FROM ME TO YOU

Advice on the Care of Your
African-American Child
Ages Birth to Twelve Months

Ena M. Cade, MD, FAAP
http://www.drcadecares.com

Disclaimer: The information presented in this book is not a substitute for medical care from a licensed healthcare provider. Please do not make any modifications, initiate or terminate any treatments without first consulting with your child's healthcare provider.

ISBN 978-0-6151-3646-2

Copyright 2006, Ena M. Cade, MD, FAAP

All rights reserved. Except as permitted under the United States Copyright Act of 1976, no part of this publication may be reproduced or distributed in any form or by any means without prior written permission of the author.

http://www.drcadecares.com

To Cebeze and Chunk

Mes raisons d'etre

CONTENTS

PREFACE	***9***
INTRODUCTION	***13***
PLANNING YOUR PREGNANCY	***19***
HEALTHY LIVING	22
SPECIFIC LIFESTYLE CHANGES	24
Smoking	24
Alcohol	26
Medications	27
Illicit drugs	28
GENERAL HEALTH	28
Age	28
Weight	29
CHRONIC MEDICAL CONDITIONS	29
Diabetes	30
High blood pressure	31
Sickle cell anemia	32
Asthma	33
Lupus	33
Sarcoidosis	34
Uterine fibroids	35
Depression	36
INFECTIOUS DISEASES	38
Gonorrhea and Chlamydia	39
Hepatitis B	39
Syphilis	40
Rubella	43
Group B Streptococcus	43
Bacterial vaginosis	44
Trichomoniasis	44
HIV	45
Herpes	47
Toxoplasmosis	48
Listeriosis	48
Chickenpox	49
PREPARING FOR BABY	***51***
CRIB SAFETY	53
CAR SAFETY	55
BABY NECCESSITIES	58
Sleeping	58

Changing diapers	*59*
General supplies	*61*
Strollers and Carriers	*65*
Toys	*66*
Feeding supplies	*70*
CHOOSING A HEALTHCARE PROVIDER	73
MD or DO	*75*
General Pediatrics or Family Medicine	*76*
Nurse Pracitioner or Physician Assistant	*77*
FEEDING YOUR BABY	78
Breastfeeding	*79*
Formula Feeding	*83*
SUPPORT SYSTEM	86

WELCOME TO THE WORLD, LITTLE ONE — 91

TYPES OF DELIVERY	93
Vaginal birth	*93*
Assisted vaginal birth	*93*
Caesarean birth	*94*
PROBLEMS DURING THE NEWBORN PERIOD	94
Prematurity	*95*
Post-maturity	*96*
Low blood-sugar	*97*
Infection	*98*
Jaundice	*99*
HOSPITAL STAY	102
In the delivery room	*102*
Baby's first 24 hours	*105*
Baby's second 24 hours	*107*

THE FIRST FEW WEEKS — 111

DAY-TO-DAY CARE	112
Feeding	*112*
Sleeping	*114*
Skin care	*117*
Hair care	*119*
TAKING CARE OF YOURSELF	120
Postpartum check	*121*
Postpartum depression	*122*

FIRST YEAR OF CHECK-UPS — 127

NEWBORN VISIT	131
2 MONTH OLD VISIT	137

4 MONTH OLD VISIT	149
6 MONTH OLD VISIT	156
9 MONTH OLD VISIT	165
ONE YEAR OLD VISIT	172

COMMON OCCURRENCES DURING THE FIRST YEAR — 177

HEAD, EYES, EAR, NOSE, AND THROAT	178
Caput and cephalohematoma	178
Positional molding	179
Vision	179
Subconjunctival hemorrhages	180
Narrow tear ducts	181
Conjunctivitis	182
Nevus of Ota	183
Eye color	183
Hearing	183
Ear pits and tags	184
Ear infection	185
Milia	187
Nasal congestion	187
Teething	188
Thrush	190
Baby bottle tooth decay	191
Laryngomalacia	193
CHEST AND LUNGS	194
Bronchiolitis	194
Accessory nipple	198
Breast buds	198
ABDOMEN AND DIGESTIVE SYSTEM	199
Vomiting	199
Umbilical hernia	200
Diarrhea	201
Constipation	202
Reflux	204
EXTREMITIES (ARMS AND LEGS)	206
Positional molding	206
Extra digits	207
SKIN	207
Skin color	207
Newborn rashes	210
Birth marks	212
Diaper rashes	213

Eczema	*215*
Cradle cap	*217*
Heart murmurs	*219*
HEART AND CIRCULATORY SYSTEM	219
Sickle cell anemia	*220*
G6PD Deficiency	*223*
Anemia	*225*
Lead poisoning	*228*
GENITAL SYSTEMS	231
Male	*231*
Female	*232*
Urinary tract infections	*233*
Hernia	*234*
GENERAL CONCERNS	236
Crying	*236*
Sudden infant death syndrome	*241*
Co-sleeping	*242*
Siblings	*245*
Pets	*248*
Child care	*249*
Baby-proofing	*253*
Fevers	*255*
CONCLUSION	**261**
APPENDIX A	**262**
APPENDIX B	**264**
VACCINE RECORD	**265**
REFERENCES	**267**

Note: In order to be gender-sensitive, this book will alternate between using the pronouns "he" and "she" from chapter to chapter. When a topic is specific to a boy or girl child, the words "male, female, boy, or girl" will be used

Preface

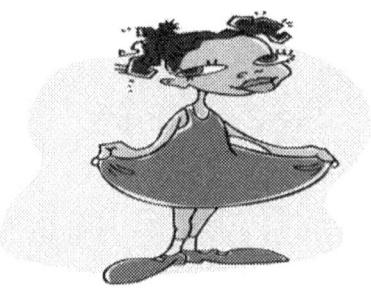

Please allow me to introduce myself. My name is Ena Marietta Cade, MD, FAAP and I am a board-certified general pediatrician. On top of that, I am the mother of two lovely boys, ages 9 months and 10 years.

Being both a mother and provider of healthcare services for infants and children, I am always drawn to the parenting section of bookstores. As an African-American woman, I have found that there are limited culturally-focused resources that address my needs and those of others like me. My goal is to create one that specifically addresses the health issues of African-American children and their families during pregnancy and the first year of life.

Throughout my medical training, I was taught the "right way" to treat and counsel patients. However, upon entering into practice, I quickly learned that often-times, there exists a rift between the "right way" and the way things are really done. Without taking the African-American culture into consideration, I would be providing a disservice to the children and families that I provide care for! Our rich history and culture inform every life decision that we make.

There are certain folk-remedies, concerns and health conditions present in the African-American community that are not necessarily present in the American community as a whole. I would like to address as many of these as possible, but no book can be all-inclusive. If you have any suggestions about sections of this book that were more or less helpful to you, as well as other topics you would have liked to have seen included, please feel free to contact me.

Thank you for your purchase of this book, and congratulations on the new addition to your family!

Introduction

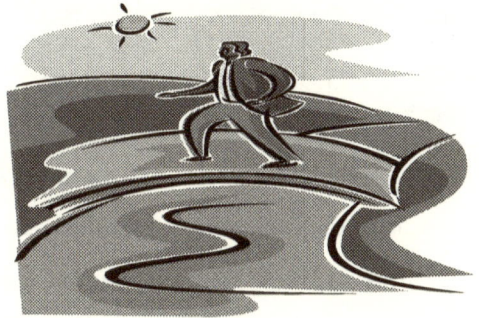

If you could decrease your baby's chance of dying from sudden infant death syndrome, would you? How about his probability of suffering from asthma, diabetes, or just being overweight in general? Unfortunately, all of these problems have much higher incidences in African-Americans. Sadder still, health disparities begin for African-Americans while they are still in the womb.[5]

The Centers for Disease Control and Prevention (CDC)'s Healthy People 2010 health survey found that the miscarriage rate for African-American women between the twentieth week of pregnancy up until delivery was 12/1000; this rate was 5/1000 in Caucasian women. Furthermore, the rate of death from all causes in infants less than one year of age was 14/1000 in African-Americans as compared with 6/1000 in Caucasians.[34]

> African-American infants are twice as likely to die before they are even born and almost **three times as likely** to die during the first year of their lives as compared with their Caucasian counterparts.

The major goal that I would like to achieve by writing this book is to bridge the gap between health and disease that exists for our children. By doing all that we can to ensure a healthy environment in which to grow, they will have better chances of living rich, full lives, and be able to contribute to society by reaching their highest potentials.

In

The

Beginning

Planning Your Pregnancy

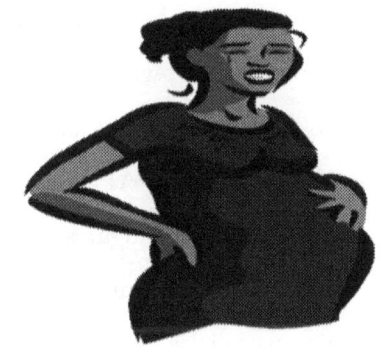

So, you have decided that you would like to have a child. This may be your first or your fourth, and each pregnancy and resulting child will be different.

Maybe in the past, you did not plan your pregnancy and you were fine, and the baby was fine, and all is well that ends well. More often than not, things probably will go well, and you may think that you need not give it a second thought. But, think about what it is that you are doing: bringing a life into this world. Through planning on your part, your baby will have a strong foundation from which to grow and prosper throughout life.

Ideally, you should schedule a pre-conception appointment with your obstetric provider. Make sure that you are up to date with all regular health screenings (PAP test, gynecologic exam, blood pressure, blood sugar and cholesterol levels, etc). Discuss the optimal nutrition and exercise programs to follow.

> If you have been using contraception, speak with your healthcare provider regarding how long it may take to be able to conceive after discontinuing the method. This will help to avoid frustration if you do not get pregnant on the first try!

Planning Your Pregnancy

If you have any long-term health issues, such as diabetes, high blood pressure or sickle-cell anemia, find out what you can do to assure a healthy start for your baby. These conditions and several others will be discussed later in this chapter.

Finally, stop your intake of alcohol. If you are a smoker, find a way to quit. By doing these things before your child is conceived, you will be ahead of the game, because you will be able to prevent exposures to your baby.

> Ask your healthcare provider to teach you how to track your menstrual cycle in order to determine the most likely time that ovulation will occur. In that way, you can "concentrate your efforts" more efficiently.

Healthy Living

Okay, now you are pregnant. Perhaps you were able to plan this pregnancy, as discussed above. Maybe you did not plan this pregnancy, but here you are, and the countdown is on!

Many women do not find out that they are pregnant until well into the first few months of pregnancy or what is called medically the first trimester. Pregnancy is broken down into three trimesters. The first one encompasses weeks one through twelve of pregnancy, and it is during this time that the foundations of the major organ systems are formed.

The importance of the first trimester cannot be understated. Any "insults," or toxins, infections, etc., to the developing baby during this crucial period could have devastating results. It is for this reason that women of childbearing age need to lead the healthiest lifestyles possible.

The definition of healthy living seems to change daily. What was exalted as a must for good health last week is now supposedly the thing that needs to be completely eliminated from your life today. Rather than change your life drastically

Planning Your Pregnancy

with each new report that comes out, stick with the tried and true basics: eat well and exercise.

Eating well includes consuming a variety of foods in order that all of your nutritional needs are met. Whenever possible, bake and steam meats and fish. Eat a wide range of vegetables of varying colors and include fruits. Limit intake of greasy, fatty foods, or what are sometimes called "empty calories." These foods contain very few, if any, nutrients and are high in fat and calories. Getting into healthy eating habits and choices now can help you to make better food decisions during pregnancy when the cravings hit.

The March of Dimes, an organization committed to the prevention of birth defects, recommends that women of childbearing age obtain at least 400 micrograms of folic acid a day from their diets.[15] This amount has been shown to significantly reduce the incidence of certain birth defects affecting the back and spine.

> Folic acid can be found in a multivitamin and is also present naturally in green leafy vegetables, enriched grains, beans, and oranges and orange juice.

Finally, stay active! Exercise does not need to consist of a formal trip to the gym. Take walks during the day, either during your lunch-break or in the morning by parking further from work than usual and walking the rest of the way (but be safe). Try evening walks with the family after dinner. These can be excellent opportunities for everyone to catch-up on each other's lives. By entering into a safe, active lifestyle now, you can continue throughout pregnancy (with your obstetrical provider's permission, of course).

Specific Lifestyle Changes
Smoking

"Smoking is not good for you" is the under-statement of the year! There are both physical (accumulation of tar in the lungs, future lung cancer, staining of the teeth, bad personal odor) and emotional (tobacco addiction) side effects to cigarette smoking.

A woman who smokes during pregnancy exposes her developing baby to the side effects of cigarette smoke as well. Smoking can lead to babies born with low birth weights. These babies have a whole host of problems, including low blood sugar levels shortly after delivery. An extended period of low blood sugar levels in an infant can cause brain damage and later learning problems.

> Infants born to mothers who smoked during pregnancy are at increased risk of dying from sudden infant death syndrome (SIDS)

For some women, pregnancy provides the last bit of inspiration needed to quit. However, the stress of caring for a newborn can cause an ex-smoker to return to cigarettes for the relief that she once received from them. Speak with your medical provider regarding support groups and other methods to help you. In particular, inquire into support groups that are designed specifically for pregnant women who are trying to quit smoking and stay off of cigarettes for good.

> The Surgeon General of the United States of America has recently released a statement regarding secondhand smoke, and no level of exposure is safe. This smoke contains over 250 chemicals that are known to be toxic to the body.[42]

Alcohol

Alcohol is an absolute "no" during pregnancy. Alcohol use during pregnancy can lead to the development of "fetal alcohol spectrum disorders." These disorders range from problems with the baby's growth during pregnancy, hyperactivity and learning disabilities, all of the way up to the fetal alcohol syndrome.[29] Fetal alcohol syndrome is associated with abnormal facial features and heart defects. There has been no safe limit determined for alcohol consumption during pregnancy; therefore, it is best to avoid it all together.

Medications

Before taking any medication (prescribed or over the counter) verify with your obstetric medical provider that it is safe. This also holds true for any natural or herbal remedies. The active ingredients in some of these remedies may be harmful to your developing baby.

Medications are classified into pregnancy drug categories that reflect the safety of their use during pregnancy. It is imperative that your treating medical provider be made aware of your pregnancy and that you find out what pregnancy class any prescribed medication is located in.

Pregnancy Medication Classifications[53]

X: Do not use during pregnancy

D: Risk of damage to developing baby

C: Risk of damage to developing baby uncertain

B: No evidence of risk in animals

A: Studies in humans show no risk

Illicit Drugs

Unfortunately, there is a long list of illicit drugs available to people who desire to use them. Each of these drugs exerts a negative effect on a developing baby. Many of these effects are life-long. If you are using any of these drugs, there is a chance that you may be addicted; PLEASE seek help, for your baby's sake and your own.

General Health

The outcome of your pregnancy is greatly influenced by your general medical condition. Extremes of age and weight are associated with specific negative outcomes during pregnancy. Both are outlined below.

Age

Younger women (aged 15 years and younger) are more likely to deliver underweight children. They also have an increased risk of developing pre-eclampsia. This is a pregnancy emergency that often requires immediate delivery of the baby. Older women (aged 35 years and older) are at an

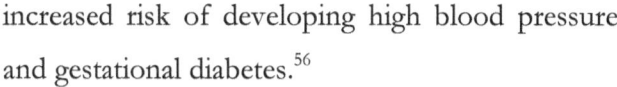 *Planning Your Pregnancy*

increased risk of developing high blood pressure and gestational diabetes.[56]

Weight

Underweight women, and those less than 100 pounds, are more likely to have underweight children. Obese women are more likely to give birth to large babies. These large babies may develop problems during and directly after birth, including difficult delivery due to size.[56]

Chronic Medical Conditions

Many chronic medical conditions can affect a growing baby. Pregnant women with these diseases are considered to have high-risk pregnancies and require close monitoring.

The Mayo Clinic suggests a preconception appointment for all women with long-term health problems.[55] This allows the woman's healthcare provider to help her prepare for the physical and emotional aspects of a high-risk pregnancy. Ideally, a chronic condition should be under the best possible control before a woman becomes pregnant. Realistically, this does not happen often.

Diabetes

Diabetes is an abnormality in which the body does not properly utilize glucose (sugar) in the bloodstream. The breakdown and storage of sugar are complex processes. The principal hormone involved is insulin. Insulin causes glucose to be taken up by the body's muscle cells and liver.

> When glucose levels are high and uncontrolled for long periods of time, damage occurs to many of the body's organs including the eyes, blood vessels and kidneys.

There are two types of diabetes that can be found in men and women. Type-one diabetes occurs when the body destroys its own insulin-producing cells. Type-two diabetes results when the body produces enough insulin but becomes resistant to its effects. This type is associated with obesity. In both types of diabetes, the end result is that the body cannot properly utilize blood glucose and its levels remain high.

Planning Your Pregnancy

Another form of diabetes, gestational diabetes, can occur in pregnant women. This condition is tested for during the second trimester of pregnancy. All three forms of diabetes can cause problems during pregnancy. These problems can include miscarriage, birth defects and over-sized babies. These babies can be difficult to deliver and may have problems with their blood sugar levels in the time period immediately following birth

> Oftentimes, children born to mothers with poorly controlled diabetes need to be cared for in a neonatal intensive care unit. The CDC recommends that a woman with diabetes try her best to plan her pregnancy and to closely monitor her blood sugar levels to keep them in the normal range.[58]

High Blood Pressure

High blood pressure can be present before, or develop during, pregnancy. It affects the developing baby by decreasing blood flow to the placenta. This in turn robs the baby of some of the oxygen and nutrients needed to grow normally.

If you have pre-existing high blood pressure, discuss the medications that you are taking with your healthcare provider. Some may have dangerous effects on your baby, and may need to be changed during your pregnancy.[56]

Sickle Cell Anemia

Having this disorder requires that you be monitored closely during pregnancy, as certain complications could arise. Among these complications is an increased risk of infections, including those of the lungs, urine, and uterus.[56]

Thirty percent of pregnant women with sickle-cell disease may develop high blood pressure, sickle-cell pain crises, stroke, and slow growth-rate of the developing baby.

> Sickle-cell anemia is present in about one out of every 500 African-Americans in the United States of America.[47]

Asthma

Not all women with asthma will experience problems during pregnancy. About half of all pregnant women with asthma do not experience any change in their asthma symptoms and, in fact, one-forth even see an improvement![56] The concern is the one-forth who develop a worsening of their symptoms. Poorly controlled asthma during pregnancy is associated with a decrease in oxygen delivered to the developing baby, thereby interfering with growth.

Notify your medical care provider immediately if you notice that your asthma symptoms are worsening. If you are pregnant during the flu season, then the flu vaccine is an absolute must. Both pregnancy and asthma increase the chances of becoming seriously ill from the flu.

Lupus

Lupus falls under the category of "autoimmune diseases." Simply stated, the body's immune system attacks itself. One of the major risk factors for the development of this disease is African-American ethnicity.

Almost 1 in every 250 African-American women has lupus. African-American women are more likely to develop lupus at younger ages and to have more serious complications from the illness.[50] Depending on the part of the body that is affected, different signs and symptoms will appear.

Complications associated with pregnancy in women who have lupus include high blood pressure, miscarriage, and neonatal lupus (a temporary condition in the baby lasting 3-6 months only).

Half of all babies born to women with lupus will have a heart condition. This heart condition has no cure, but it can be successfully managed with a pacemaker to control the baby's heart rate.

Sarcoidosis

Sarcoidosis is a disease that is not very well understood. Inflammation and then scarring occurs in various organs of the body. Symptoms are related to the organs involved.

Planning Your Pregnancy

Sarcoidosis is more common in African-American women, particularly those between the ages of 20 and 40 years.[48] Most of the medications used to treat this disease are dangerous for use during pregnancy. For this reason, let your healthcare provider know immediately if you become or are planning to become pregnant, in order that necessary adjustments can be made to your treatment regimen.

Uterine Fibroids

Uterine fibroids are non-cancerous tumors that can be found in the uterus. African-American women are two to three times more likely to suffer symptoms from fibroids, and these fibroids are also more likely to appear at an earlier age. If the fibroids are large enough, they can interfere with implantation of a fertilized egg, growth of the baby due to space constraints and delivery due to physical blockage of the cervix.[56]

> If you have a history of uterine fibroids, discuss this with your doctor. They can be easily evaluated by ultrasound examination of the uterus.

Depression

Studies have shown that 10-20% of women will have depression during pregnancy.[58] Sadly, there is still a stigma that exists when it comes to mental illness. This stigma may be even more prevalent in African-American communities, with some people going without treatment due to the belief that depression is a sign of personal weakness. Depression can be treated and improves quality of life for both the individual and his or her family.

Women who have depression will oftentimes face a dilemma when they decide to have a baby. There is not much hard data to support the use of anti-depressant medications in pregnant women. There are some medications that are known to cause problems during pregnancy and are to be avoided; however, there are others that appear to be safe.

In cases of severe depression, the benefits of treating the mother far outweigh the possible risks to the developing baby. Untreated depression during pregnancy can lead to the mother having a decreased ability to care for herself as well as an increase in the likelihood of the use of substances that endanger her developing baby (e.g. alcohol, cigarettes, illicit drugs).[68]

If you have depression, speak with your treating provider regarding your medications and what you should do during your pregnancy. DO NOT stop your medications without your healthcare provider's knowledge.

> Severe, untreated depression has a negative effect on pregnancy by decreasing blood flow across the placenta to the baby and leads to premature birth and low birth weight.[68]

Infectious Diseases

Several infectious diseases have been recognized as causing serious problems in infants. Some of these infectious diseases are routinely screened for when a woman receives prenatal care. Others, however, are not routine tests. It is up to you to know what your risk factors are and to discuss them with your healthcare provider.

I have outlined below many of the infectious diseases that could have a negative impact on your growing baby. I strongly urge you to speak candidly with your healthcare provider regarding any sexually transmitted infections that you have had in the past. This will help him or her to decide whether further tests or precautions during your baby's delivery are needed.

Routine Tests

A routine test is one that is done on every person who presents to the medical care provider's office. For a pregnant woman, these tests include those for gonorrhea, chlamydia, hepatitis B, syphilis, rubella and group B streptococcus.

Gonorrhea and Chlamydia

These are both sexually transmitted infections that can be passed on to an infant during the birthing process. Most women are checked for gonorrhea and chlamydia during their yearly gynecological exams. It is important to know that either of these infections could be present in a woman who has no symptoms at all.

In newborns, both infections can cause eye infections, with an especially severe form caused by gonorrhea. Chlamydia can also cause pneumonia and gonorrhea, meningitis (a serious brain infection).[41] These infections can be easily treated with antibiotics taken by the mother during pregnancy.

Hepatitis B

Hepatitis is the general term for inflammation of the liver. It can be caused by many different entities, including alcohol, some drugs and infections.

Of particular concern during pregnancy is hepatitis due to the hepatitis B virus. This virus can be passed to babies from infected mothers, so the presence or absence of the infection must be determined well in advance of delivery. If a mother is known to be infected with hepatitis B then her baby can receive two important vaccines right in the delivery room.

According to the American Academy of Pediatrics (AAP)'s Red Book of Infectious Diseases in Children, **95%** of transmissions of hepatitis B from mother to baby can be prevented if early vaccinations are given![12] 90% of babies who do become infected at the time of birth will go on to develop chronic hepatitis B infection. This carries with it a greatly increased risk of liver cancer.[12]

Syphilis

Syphilis is caused by an organism called a spirochete. Women are tested for syphilis at least once during pregnancy and some medical practitioners will check again at around the time of delivery.

Infected mothers pass the spirochete to their developing babies. Babies born with syphilis infections develop problems with bone growth, the skin and liver. If not detected early and then treated, the disease will pass through several different stages and eventually affect the heart and nervous system.[8]

Syphilis is treated with penicillin, which the mother can receive during pregnancy. An infected baby can receive this medication right after birth to prevent any further damage to his or her system.

The Tuskegee Experiment[59]

When referring to syphilis, its medical course, and treatment, one would be remiss to leave out a discussion of the infamous "Tuskegee Experiment." The medical profession owes much of what it knows about syphilis to 400 African-American sharecroppers from Macon County, Alabama. These men were enrolled in a study in which they were denied treatment for syphilis. The study was in effect from 1932-1972, and a known, effective treatment (penicillin) was available in 1947. The men were never told that they had syphilis, but rather "bad blood." They were offered "treatments" that were actually tests done to follow the evolution of the syphilis infection. The study ended in 1972 when a sexually transmitted infections investigator, Peter Buxtun, alerted the media.

Rubella

Rubella, also known as German measles, has devastating effects on a developing baby when the mother is infected during pregnancy. These effects include deafness, heart and eye abnormalities and nervous system defects.

The rubella vaccine has been a recommended childhood vaccination for some years now. Occasionally, however, a woman is found to not have immunity to this virus. In such a case, the vaccine will be given before she leaves the hospital after delivery. It is not advised to give the vaccine during pregnancy nor to become pregnant within 28 days of receiving it.[13]

Group B Streptococcus

This bacterium, which is not known to be a sexually transmitted infection, rarely causes problems in the mother; she is simply in what is called a "carrier state" whereby the bacteria are present in the vaginal and rectal areas and, occasionally, the urine.

In a newborn infant, group B streptococcus can cause severe and sometimes fatal infections including pneumonia and meningitis.[9] Detection of these bacteria is simple, involving only a cotton-swabbed specimen of the vagina and rectum. The test should be done between the 35th and 37th weeks of pregnancy. Treatment consists of giving the mother antibiotics during delivery.

Non-Routine Tests

These are all tests that will be done on an as-needed basis. "As-needed" can be due to symptoms of possible infection, such as a vaginal discharge, or due to risk, such as HIV. Even though not routine, I highly recommend that all pregnant women be tested for the presence of HIV antibodies (commonly known as the "HIV test").

Bacterial Vaginosis

This is a condition in which certain bacteria normally present in the vagina overgrow. The infection is usually associated with an itchy discharge and is diagnosed by examining the vaginal discharge with the aid of a microscope.

Bacterial vaginosis should be treated as its presence is associated with premature labor and delivery.[41]

Trichomoniasis

This is a sexually transmitted infection that, like bacterial vaginosis, can lead to premature labor if not treated. The infection is caused by an organism called a protozoa and can also be diagnosed by microscopic examination of the vaginal discharge.

After treatment, all towels and personal garments should be washed well in hot water and dried on a high setting. Trichomonads can live on towels and cause re-infection or be passed to a household member.[41]

HIV

HIV infections are increasing at an alarming rate in African-American women. According to the Centers for Disease Control and Prevention (CDC), in the year 2002 AIDS was the leading cause of death for African American women aged 25-34 years. Based on the statistics from 2004, **78%** of all new HIV infections were due to heterosexual contact. Even more alarming, of the 123,405 women living with HIV/AIDS, **64%** were African-American.[25]

A woman with HIV can be treated during pregnancy and delivery, deliver her child by caesarean section and her baby be treated for a few months afterwards with medications to help prevent transmission of the virus. The effectiveness rate of this process is an almost 85% reduction in transmission of HIV from mother to infant.[15]

> If you are pregnant then you were possibly exposed to HIV. Knowing your HIV status before delivery could be the difference between passing the virus onto your child or not.

Herpes

Herpes is an extremely common infection. It is estimated that 45 million Americans are carriers of this virus.[41] Herpes viruses are actually in the same class as varicella viruses, the virus that causes chickenpox. These viruses remain in the nerves of the affected body part and can reactivate at any time, usually during times of illness or stress.

The concern with herpes infection is whether or not the disease is active at the time of delivery. The initial herpes infection, called the primary infection, is usually painful and easy to detect. However, reoccurrences can be mild and sometimes are not noticed at all.

Some obstetricians prefer to deliver a woman with genital herpes by caesarean section in order to prevent passage of the virus to the baby during a vaginal birth. Herpes infection in a newborn infant is devastating and can lead to death.

Other Infections

Toxoplasmosis

Toxoplasma are parasites found in cat feces, soil and raw or undercooked meats. If a woman is infected during pregnancy, her growing baby can develop problems with the brain, eyes and liver.[14]

If you have cats, relegate the litter-changing duties to another family member. If you absolutely must be the one to change the litter, wear gloves and wash your hands well afterwards. In addition, avoid eating raw or undercooked meats.

Listerisosis

Listeria are bacteria that can cause miscarriage as well as meningitis in the newborn child.[10] Listeria can be found in unpasteurized milk (especially goats' milk), soft cheese (feta, brie), undercooked meats and unwashed fresh produce. Be sure to cook all meats thoroughly, wash all vegetables before consumption and avoid the foods listed above. Thankfully, this infection is

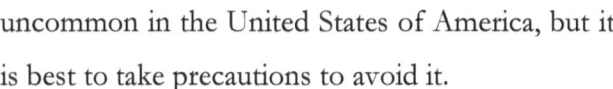

uncommon in the United States of America, but it is best to take precautions to avoid it.

Chickenpox

Most adults have been exposed to varicella, the virus that causes chickenpox, at some time or other during childhood or adolescence. Unfortunately, there are some who are not immune to this virus either because they were never exposed or had a very mild infection that did not trigger immunity in their bodies.

The effects of varicella virus infection on a developing baby will depend on the stage of pregnancy in which it occurs. These effects can include abnormal development of the arms and legs, scarring of the skin and eye defects.[11] Avoid contact with any children who have fevers or rashes to be on the safe side.

Preparing for Baby

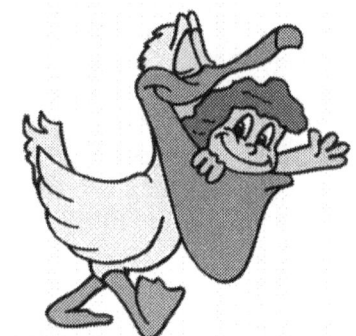

Parents put much thought and enthusiasm into the color scheme and theme of their soon-to-arrive baby's room. Picking out the crib with a matching changing table, dresser and wall appliqués can be quite exciting!

From Me To You

Always have safety in mind as you prepare this special part of your home. Your baby's room is where she will spend much of her time, not just sleeping, but playing and exploring. In addition to your baby's room, your entire home will be utilized in one way or another during your day-to-day care of the baby.

This chapter focuses on preparing your home for your little one's arrival and will identify many of the safety issues that need to be addressed when doing so. In addition to in your own home, be sure to get everyone on board with your child's safety preparations. This includes all relatives who will be caring for your baby, as their homes need to be scrutinized in the same manner that you do your own.

A commonly encountered response to new parents requesting that certain things be done with their babies is "we did it this way with you, and you turned out fine." There is an excellent link on the Consumer Product Safety Commission (CPSC)'s web site for grandparents and other caretakers who may not agree with some of the childcare recommendations of today.[33] This link

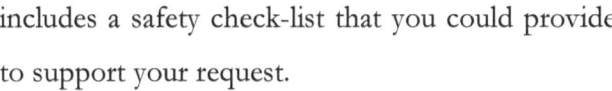 *Preparing For Baby*

includes a safety check-list that you could provide to support your request.

Crib Safety

Cribs vary in color, finish, even size and shape. However, all new cribs must meet the regulations of the Consumer Product Safety Commission (CPSC) of the United States Government. This commission is charged with the task of maintaining that regulations are in place to assure that the products we are sold are safe when used in the manner intended. In addition, the CPSC issues recalls of products that are found to be unsafe after they have been released on the market.

Please know that older or "heirloom" cribs will likely not meet the guidelines outlined by the CPSC for crib safety. They also may contain lead-based paints which your baby will consume when she chews on the bars (as teething babies often do). If there is an heirloom crib in your home and your family insists on your using it, because you and every other person in the family slept in it, do not be afraid to say no. Just explain that you

From Me To You

would like to experience the joy of picking out your own furniture for the baby.

The following are recommendations for crib safety as outlined by the Consumer Product Safety Commission:[60]

- ଔ There should be no gaps between the mattress and the crib's edges (to prevent the head from becoming trapped in the little space that could be created).

- ଔ No lose or missing hardware (screws, etc).

- ଔ No more than 2 3/8 inches between the crib bars. Any larger and your baby's body could fit through.

- ଔ No corner posts over 1/16th inch high. Baby's clothes could become caught, causing strangulation.

- ଔ No cutout patterns in the head or footboards Baby's head could become trapped.

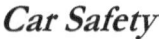   *Preparing For Baby*

Car Safety

In many states, parents cannot leave the hospital with their new baby without demonstrating that they have an appropriate infant car seat <u>and</u> know how to use it.

When choosing a car seat, it is recommended that unless you are absolutely certain of the seat's accident history, do not buy a used one. Even if the seat appears to be in good repair, a car seat that has been involved in a car crash should not be used for transporting your infant.

The National Highway Transportation Safety Administration (NHTSA) has recently modified its recommendations regarding car seats involved in car crashes.[49] Their position is that child restraints that have been in minor crashes do not need to be replaced, and can be re-used.

> There are five criteria that need to be met in order for a car crash to be classified as "minor." My recommendation would be to err on the side of safety and purchase a new seat.

55

When using a car seat for an infant, remember to always use the harness system to secure the child in place. Unfortunately, people sometimes forget to do that, or think it is not necessary if the child is just sitting on the floor in the seat. Car seats can topple over or parents can pick the car seat up without remembering to re-secure the baby with the harnesses. Never leave the car seat on a high surface (table or countertop) from which it could fall, or on a soft surface (such as a bed), on which it can topple over and suffocate the baby.

Infants aged birth through 1 year and under 20 pounds should ride in an infant-only or convertible seat in the rear-facing position. An infant this age and size does not have the neck control to support the head in the front-facing position should a crash occur. The safest place for a baby to ride in a car is the rear middle seat. Never place the baby in a front seat if there is an air-bag present. Once the infant weighs over 20 pounds but is still under one year of age, a convertible seat may be used, but still placed in the rear-facing position.

All car seats come with a piece called a locking clip, which serves to anchor the seat in place. Newer cars come with a LATCH car-seat attachment system; this system allows for the car-seat to be attached directly to the automobile's frame with a special hook and belt. Once properly installed, you should not be able to move the car seat more than one inch from side-to-side.

> An infant seat is one that is made for use by infants only, i.e. children less than 12 months of age. The upper weight limit for these seats generally ranges from 20 to 22 pounds.
>
> A convertible seat is one that can be used for infants or children. These seats must be used in the rear-facing position for any child less than 12 months of age.

Baby Necessities

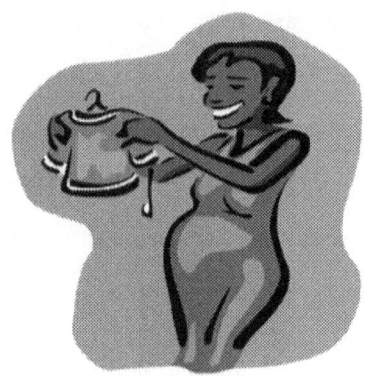

There is an entire market targeted towards the soft hearts of new parents. I will present you with the basics that are needed for the first few months at home with your baby. The decision between primary or pastel colors is left to you!

Place to sleep

Your baby will spend most of the first few months of her life sleeping. Although it is exciting to pick out a crib, many parents find that they do not even use this piece of furniture during the baby's first weeks at home.

For nighttime convenience, you may want to purchase a bassinette or other small, safe sleeping space for your baby. If you will be breastfeeding, it is easier to have the baby close by, not down the hall in a separate nursery. Consider purchasing a soft night-light, so that you do not illuminate the entire room when feeding or changing your baby at night.

Place to change diapers

A complete nursery furniture set usually includes a matching changing table. While it may be attractive, the truth of the matter is that you will most likely change your baby in whatever spot she is in when she needs changing. A good investment is a portable, washable changing pad that will offer protection when the baby is changed on an area you want to keep clean (bed, sofa).

Remember, never leave your baby unattended on any surface, as she may roll off and become injured. If you do purchase a changing table, do not be lulled into a false sense of security when you use the straps to secure your baby in place.

> Assemble everything you need (or think you may need) before starting to change the baby. That way, it will not be necessary to step away or turn your back on her while she is on the changing table.

Place to bathe

Many parents find an infant bathing basin to be a convenience. Some basins come with a sling which will support your baby in a lying position as you bathe her. Others grow with your baby, and include a support seat for when she can sit unassisted.

Never leave your baby unattended in the tub, even if she seems well supported and there is only an inch of water in the tub or basin. Children can drown very quickly, and no phone call or forgotten bathing supply is worth your child's life. If you must go retrieve something during baby's bath time, wrap her up in a towel and take her with you.

Preparing For Baby

Baby Supplies

BATHING

- Mild, tear-free bathing wash
- Rubbing alcohol (for umbilical cord care)
- Diaper rash cream
    - Baby powder is not recommended, as the dust from the powder can enter the baby's lungs and cause pneumonia.
- Baby oil or lotion
- Cotton balls
    - Cotton swabs are not recommended, as they can injure the ear-drum.
- Baby towels and washcloths
- Infant comb and brush

CLOTHING

- One-piece underwear
- Sleep sacks
    - These are excellent to use in place of blankets. Blankets are not recommended for use in newborn and young infants, as they may inadvertently slide up over the baby's face.

- Weather appropriate outfits
  - The number of outfits that you purchase is up to you. Your baby may go through two or three outfits in one day, depending on whether or not she spits-up a lot or has loose bowel-movements that run through her diaper.
  - If your child is born in the winter, have appropriate clothing for cold weather. It is better to dress the baby in layers, which can easily be added or removed should she become too cold or hot.
  - In the summer, be careful to not overdress the baby. For the first few months, a baby's heat control system is not well developed. She will have trouble releasing excess heat through sweat and run the risk of overheating.
- Mild laundry detergent

GENERAL SUPPLIES

- Diapers

  ~ In the early newborn period, you may want to purchase diapers that have a "cut-out" area for the healing umbilical cord.

  > **Cloth Diapers**
  >
  > Some families are choosing to use cloth diapers. Cloth diapers have come a long way from the times of pins and rubber pants. There are many companies that you can find on the web that sell cloth diapers with Velcro® closures, absorbable liners and even cute patterns that offer some variety to your baby's wardrobe.

- Wipes

  ~ You can always use a cloth moistened with warm water to clean your baby. I recommend that babies be cleaned after each change diaper, even if they were only wet.

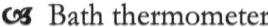

- ෬ Bath thermometer
  - ~ The thermometer is placed in the water, and displays the safe temperature zone for your baby's bath.

BEDDING

- ෬ Fitted sheets made specifically for cribs. Loose-fitting sheets can allow for extra material to puff-out, resulting in a suffocation hazard.
- ෬ No stuffed toys If you have them, keep them out of the crib. The baby could bury her face in one and suffocate.
- ෬ No comforters or blankets
- ෬ No pillows
  - ~ Many stores sell baby pillows, but these should be for decoration only.
- ෬ Bumpers
  - ~ There is a chance of entrapment between the bumper and the crib rails. If you do use a bumper, remove it once the baby is able to roll over or push up on her knees.

ༀ Crib mattress.

  ~ The mattress must be the appropriate size for the crib you will be using, in order that there will be no gaps that the baby's head could become trapped in.

Transportation Outside of the Car

Strollers

To prevent injuries to your baby from the stroller tipping over, The Juvenile Products Manufacturers Association (JPMA) recommends the purchase of a wide-based stroller. In addition, assure that it will not flip backwards if you lie your baby back in the reclining position.

Carriers

When choosing a carrier for your infant, ask around to find recommendations from friends and family. There are so many choices available to you that this could help to narrow down your selection.

As with all else, safety should be the first priority in making your choice. Regardless of the

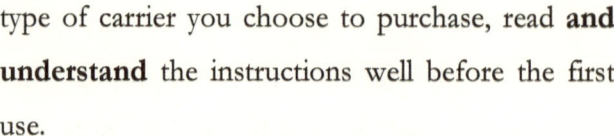

type of carrier you choose to purchase, read **and understand** the instructions well before the first use.

Toys

The market for infant toys is enormous and the target-age range has now expanded to include babies still in the womb! Books, stuffed animals, mobiles: the variety can seem endless and overwhelming.

First and foremost, be sure that the toys you purchase are safe and age-appropriate. By the time your baby is 4 months old, everything that she gets in her hands will go straight to her mouth. Choking is a great hazard, and also needs to be considered if there is an older sibling in the home with toys that may be to small for the baby.

The next thing to consider is your baby's developmental stage. Immediately after birth, infants can see about as far as the distance of your forearm's length. Infants at this age prefer geometric shapes in black-and white and human faces.

Between about the 4th and 5th months, many infants enjoy having toys dangle in front of them. There are toys available that will make noises or play music when pulled by the baby

> Never use a string to tie a toy to your baby to play with, as this poses a strangulation hazard.

As your baby learns how to pull herself up to stand, she may enjoy toys that allow her to pull up and "cruise" around the edges. Oftentimes these toys are adorned with different shapes, colors, mirrors and music to amuse your curious baby.

Finally, once your baby is beginning to take some steps, there are toys that she can push around like a cart. Just make sure that they do not roll too quickly, as the baby may fall forward and hurt her face!

Many babies also enjoy bearing weight on their legs and bouncing up and down. There is a wide-range of toys available that will support your baby's weight while she bounces. Be sure that the product you use is stationary. The American Academy of Pediatrics (AAP) has issued a statement that the use of walkers should be banned.

> The American Academy of Pediatrics has recommended a ban on the manufacture and sale of infant walkers in the United States.[5]
>
> Research has shown that walkers do not, contrary to popular belief, strengthen a baby or improve her walking; children who have spent time in walkers sit, crawl, and walk later than children not spending time in walkers.
>
> Walkers also allow infants easier access to hazards such as stoves and poisons. If you do decide to use a walker, buy one that is certified by the Juvenile Products Manufacturers Association (JPMA) and that complies with standard ASTM-F077-96.

Often overlooked as toys for children, books are essential for helping your baby to develop many necessary skills. Begin to introduce books to your child at around the age of six months. You will notice that books made for infants this age are constructed of thick cardboard which will withstand all of the sucking and chewing that a baby does.

While reading a book to your baby, point out the colors, make sounds that correspond to the animals or other characters present and just have fun! If you can't get past the second page, don't worry. Your baby has a very short attention span at this age. Be prepared for some well-meaning folks to tell you that reading to a baby is silly. But, don't let it stop you! You really are your child's first teacher. The more you do to provide stimulation to her now, the more benefits she will reap later.

> **Television and Babies**
>
> The American Academy of Pediatrics recommends that television be <u>completely avoided</u> during the first two years of a child's life. They point out that infants achieve optimal brain development during this stage of life through direct interaction with their caregivers.[56]

Feeding Supplies

Whether you have decided to breast or bottle feed, there are some common supplies that you should have on hand at home.

For mothers who have decided to breastfeed, investing in a good breast-pump is essential if they plan to spend any time away from their babies. Look-up reviews of different breast-pumps on web sites for breastfeeding support organizations such as La Leche League or the African-American Breastfeeding Alliance. Ask any friends who have breastfed for their input as well.

The type of pump you may need will depend on the frequency of pumping necessary. For intermittent use, a hand pump may suffice; for mothers who are returning to work, a higher-grade, electric pump, perhaps one with double-pumping action, might be more appropriate due to its time saving advantages.

If you have decided to bottle-feed, then purchase enough bottles and nipples to cover an entire day's feedings. It may be convenient to prepare the bottles beforehand and store them in the refrigerator.

> Never reheat milk in a microwave. Microwaves heat foods unevenly, creating hot pockets that will burn your baby's mouth In addition microwaving actually destroys many of the healthy components present in breast milk.

Until the baby is about six months of age, you should sterilize her bottles, nipples and basically all else that goes into her mouth. Before that time, her immune system is still immature. Commercial sterilizers are available in almost any store where baby products are sold and range from microwavable to electronic in nature. Of course, you can always sterilize the "old-fashioned way" by boiling all bottles, nipples and pacifiers for twenty minutes.

Bibs are a must, as most infants spit-up a little milk when they burp. They also can help to prevent milk from dripping into your baby's difficult to reach neck folds. Chronic moisture in that area often leads to painful chafing, which is difficult to get rid of once it develops.

Choosing a Healthcare Provider

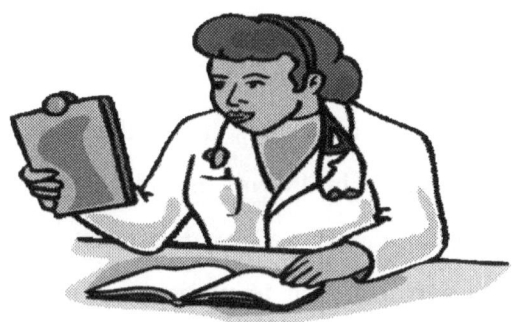

Choosing your baby's healthcare provider is not a decision to be taken lightly. This will be the person with whom you will entrust your precious child's medical care. You want to be able to have confidence in her advice and be comfortable in asking any and all questions that you may have. You should not be made to feel "bad" for wanting advice and reassurance in the early months.

Some of the best resources available for finding a healthcare provider for your child are friends and family. Find out how long it takes to get a well-baby appointment, the policies on sick-visits, usual waiting room time, what to do in case of emergency when the office is closed, and the office hours (including the availability of evening and weekend hours).

If possible, schedule a "prenatal visit", which is actually covered by many insurance companies (but check first). This will give you and your new baby's healthcare provider a chance to meet, go over your and your partner's medical histories and help you to prepare for the baby's upcoming birth and early care. Also, take the opportunity to interact with the medical office staff. Determine if you feel that you are in an comfortable environment.

Below, there are descriptions of the different types of healthcare providers that you may encounter while making your decision. This information can be used as just one part of your decision making process,. Finding the right "fit" is sometimes a process of trial and error. You will be seeing this person on a regular basis for the first two years of your child's life, so choose wisely!

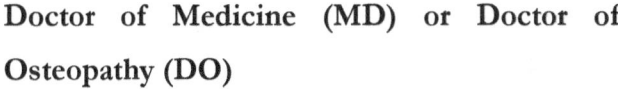

Doctor of Medicine (MD) or Doctor of Osteopathy (DO)

When choosing a physician to provide your child's medical care, you will see one of two sets of initials behind the name. There may be other initials representing other degrees, but the medical degrees are signified by MD (doctor of medicine) or DO (doctor of osteopathy).

A doctor of medicine is one who has completed a course of study approved by the Association of American Medical Colleges. This entity has established guidelines for the education and training of physicians. "MD" doctors are trained to approach the body in a "systems" manner.

A doctor of osteopathy is one who has completed training in an accredited school of osteopathic medicine. "DO" physicians are trained to view the human body as functioning as a whole, and also use manipulative treatments to realign the body.

Both types of doctors are required to complete residency training in order to become board-certified in a specialty area of patient care.

General Pediatrics or General/Family Medicine

There are two general specialties that provide care for children: pediatrics and general/family medicine.

Pediatricians complete a three-year residency program during which they participate in the care of children in the hospital and office settings. There are usually rotations through many of the pediatric sub-specialties as well (such as cardiology, endocrinology, development, and intensive care).

At the end of residency training, a physician is considered "board-eligible," which means that she can take the board examination and become board-certified. Being board-certified reflects the fact that the physician has successfully passed an exam developed by the American Board of Pediatrics that is felt to represent competency in the care of children.

Pediatricians are required to re-certify every 7 years. This ensures that they are keeping up-to-date with the ever-changing practices that may occur in their field.

Family physicians typically complete a three-year residency program of rotation through the different specialties in medicine, including internal medicine, obstetrics and gynecology, and pediatrics. Upon completion of their training, these physicians are also considered "board-eligible" and may sit for the board examination offered by the American Board of Family Medicine.

> Some physicians are double-boarded in internal medicine and pediatrics. These physicians have completed a program of training that satisfies the requirements for both the boards of pediatrics and internal medicine.

Nurse Practitioner (NP) or Physician Assistant (PA)

These medical professionals work alongside physicians to provide medical care to patients. Both have requirements for a supervising "physician of record" to co-manage patients. These requirements differ based on the state in which they practice.

Feeding Your Baby

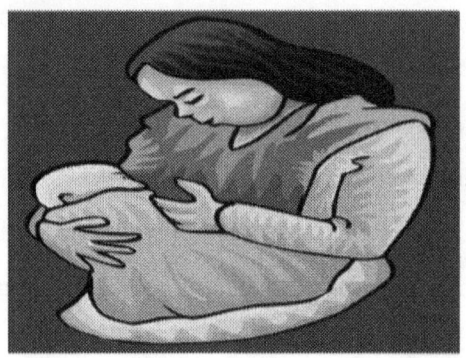

The ideal time to decide how you will feed your baby is before she is born. The choice between feeding your infant formula or breast milk is a personal one. In some families, all of the babies have been breastfed, whereas in others, all receive formula. Some women who decide that they would like to breastfeed may stop before they would have liked to because they assumed it would just come naturally when, in fact, it is a learned skill.

This section will present to you the benefits and pitfalls of each form of feeding so that you can make an informed decision. As a pediatrician, and a mother, I recommend that all infants be breastfed, exclusively (no supplements), for the first 6 months of life as recommended by the American Academy of Pediatrics.[7]

Breastfeeding

Any review of studies on infant feeding will confirm that breast milk is superior to any other form of infant feeding. The American Academy of Pediatrics issued a policy statement on breastfeeding in February 2005.[7] In it, they state that the advantages of breastfeeding "include health, nutritional, immunologic, developmental, psychological, social, economic, and environmental benefits."

The initial fluid that is present in the breasts immediately after birth, colostrum, is full of antibodies. These antibodies help to fight infections. This is essential for infants, as their immune systems are not mature until 6 months of age.

> Breastfed infants have less illness due to meningitis, ear infections, urinary tract infections, and diarrhea.[7]

There are also benefits for the breastfeeding mom. Each time a woman breastfeeds, a hormone called oxytonin is released into her bloodstream. This hormone helps the uterus to return to its pre-pregnancy size more rapidly. Studies have also shown that there is a decreased risk of breast cancer, ovarian cancer and osteoporosis.[7]

If you decide that breastfeeding is what you would like to do for you and your baby, begin early on in pregnancy with reading and learning about it. Being prepared is one of the most important steps that you can take in assuring that you are able to start and continue breastfeeding for your planned duration.

If there are women in your family or circle of friends who have breastfed, seek advice from them. Also, enquire about breastfeeding classes at the place in which you receive your prenatal care. There is a lot to learn in terms of different holding positions, Common Concerns that may arise, and where to go for help and support. Other sources of support include La Leche League, and the

African American Women's Breastfeeding Alliance (see Appendix A for contact information)

> **Composition of Breast Milk**
>
> Breast milk is described as a "species-specific, live fluid that changes from day to day."[40] The composition of breast milk changes during a feeding as well! The initial, or foremilk, has a high water content to satisfy your infant's thirst; the later, or hind-milk, is higher in fat and calories to satisfy hunger.
>
> Mature milk is composed of fats, hormones, sugars, proteins, and even white blood cells to help prevent infections! Among the fats is one called DHA, which is needed for optimal visual development.

Breastfeeding and Returning to Work

Returning to the workplace does not mean that you must put an end to breastfeeding your child. Many mothers feel a sense of pride in knowing that they are providing nourishment to their child while away from the home. They are also able to reconnect with their babies at the end of the day by having a feeding.

Essential to successful breastfeeding while working outside of the home is a reliable, efficient breast pump and some planning on your part. Review your expected daily work-routine and determine when you could take breaks to pump. You will need to find a private place, free of interruptions for about 15-20 minutes depending on the efficiency of the pump you will use. Finally, locate a safe place to store your expressed milk. Some pumps include storage bags with freezer packs to maintain freshness for up to 8 hours or so.

> In order to maintain your milk supply, try not to let more than four hours lapse between pumping sessions. While at home with your infant on weekends and evenings, continue to breastfeed on demand.

Preparing For Baby

Who Should NOT Breastfeed?

The following is a list of conditions under which a woman should not breastfeed. In addition, if you are taking any substance (even if it is over the counter, herbal, or "natural"), speak with your care provider regarding the safety of breastfeeding:[7]

- Infants with classic galactosemia
- Mothers who are positive for human T-cell lymphotrophic virus I or II
- Mothers who are HIV positive
- Mothers receiving radioactive medications
- Mothers receiving chemotherapy
- Mothers with active herpes sores on the breast
- Mothers who abuse illicit drugs

Formula Feeding

There was once a time when nearly every child was fed breast milk. This is not to say that they were breastfed by their mothers. Some families employed "wet-nurses," or women who were lactating (producing milk) to feed their infants![57] Wet-nurses would register with agencies and submit to physical examinations to assess their general health status. The agencies were then able to connect the nurses with families in need of them and allowed for certain standards to be kept in terms of quality of the milk that was being provided.

Over time, the demand for wet nurses decreased, and a breast milk substitute was needed for those women who did not, or could not, choose to breastfeed their infants. Early in the 19th century, milk from many different animals was used as human milk substitutes. Finally, in 1838, a scientist was able to analyze and report on the composition of breast milk and cow's milk. [57]

Using this information, companies began to develop infant formulas that closely approximated the composition of breast milk. Over the years, as more and more breast milk components have been discovered, modifications of infant formulas have been made. There are now infant formulas available for infants who have milk-protein allergy, reflux, and metabolic disorders that prohibit the use of breast milk.

Preparing For Baby

If you chose to formula feed your baby, begin with knowing the type of formula that you are using. Infant formulas come in ready-to-feed, concentrated liquid and powdered preparations. Ready-to-feed means just that; no preparation is needed other than to pour the formula into a bottle and add a nipple. Concentrated liquid requires dilution with water before feeding. Powder must be mixed with water before usage.

Follow the preparation instructions **exactly as outlined** by the manufacturer. Any modifications that are made (using more or less water, adding water to ready-to-feed) can have dire consequences, including the death of your baby!

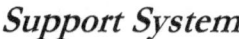

Support System

In the days and first several weeks after your child's birth, there will very little sleep accompanied by stress and overall fatigue. To expect that you can do it all, in terms of taking care of the house, preparing meals, and caring for your other children (if you have them) is unrealistic and will set you up for trouble.

> As African-American women, we sometimes become accustomed to "doing it all" without a single complaint or asking for help. It is okay to ask for and accept help! Receiving help is not a sign of personal weakness

Support comes in many forms. The most basic is physical support, which will be necessary during the first few weeks after bringing your new baby home from the hospital. Your body needs to recuperate. In addition to the physical challenges of birth, there are also hormonal changes that take place that may leave you feeling worn down. Having someone around to help out, even if only to allow you to take a much needed nap, is an invaluable resource! Ask your partner or other support person to enquire into the possibility of Family Medical Leave; fathers are entitled to paternity leave just as new mothers are to maternity leave!

If you have friends and family who are willing, ask that they prepare a meal or two that can be frozen and simply reheated at mealtime. You can also cook and safely store meals to have on stock for the days when you feel too drained to think about "what's for dinner?" let alone make it!

Finally, you may consider joining a support group. In particular, Mocha Moms is a group of African-American women who have chapters nationwide to foster sisterhood amongst mothers. Check online for the location of your local chapter (See Appendix A).

A Child Is Born

Welcome To The World, Little One

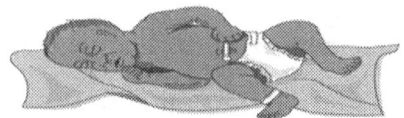

After what may have seemed to you to be an eternity of waiting, the big day has arrived! Being prepared can help to ease some of the anxiety that you may experience.

Learn as much as possible about the birthing process, perhaps through attending a Lamaze class during your pregnancy. Remember, however, that sometimes things do not go as planned. Learn about what caesarean sections (c-sections) are and what to expect should you need one.

When you leave for the hospital, don't forget to take a packed baby bag! Remember to pack a special outfit for the all-important first photo, which is usually offered by the hospital nursery. Pack some diapers, baby wipes, a change of clothes, mini changing-pad, and you are good to go!

This chapter will begin with a review of a few types of deliveries from a pediatric perspective and how they may affect your baby. I will also discuss some complications that may arise in the early newborn period. Do not focus on what may go wrong! I have included these topics in the event that your baby develops any of the more common, easily treatable conditions that can occur during his transition to life outside of your womb.

Types of Delivery

Vaginal Birth

During a vaginal delivery, the baby must be pushed, preferably head first, through the cervix, down the vaginal canal and, finally, out of the vaginal opening. Babies who are delivered after a long pushing phase of labor will likely have some misshaping of their heads. They may also develop bruising of the face and red spots in the whites of the eyes. All of these changes will resolve with time, and are not signs of any deep injury to the head, brain or eyes.

> The bones of an infant's skull are connected by soft cartilage, which allows them to overlap and mold for an easier passage out.

Assisted Vaginal Birth

Sometimes a baby needs a little help exiting. The obstetrical medical provider may decide to implement forceps or a vacuum to assist the baby out. When these devices are used, the baby may get some bruising on the temples and cheeks from forceps or at the top of the head from vacuum suction. Again, these are superficial bruises, and will resolve with time.

Caesarean Delivery

These babies are usually the ones with the perfect round little heads if the caesarean was planned and labor did not occur. A pediatrician should be present in the delivery room to examine all babies born in this manner. The reason for this is that some babies born by caesarean have trouble transitioning, or adjusting to life outside of the womb, for the first several minutes to hours after birth.

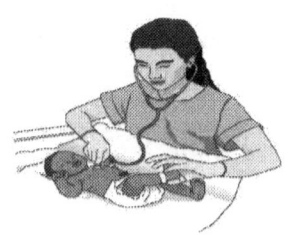

Problems During the Newborn Period

Fortunately, many of the issues that arise right after birth are easily treated when detected early. Should you have any concerns, do not be afraid to say something to your baby's nurse or other medical provider.

Prematurity

A term pregnancy is one that lasts any where from 38-42 weeks. A baby born before that time is pre-term (premature) and a baby born after, post-term.

When an infant is born pre-term, a whole host of problems may arise. A baby born at 36 weeks of pregnancy will tend to have fewer problems than a baby born at 32 weeks. Keep in mind, however, that the reason behind the premature birth will also affect a baby's outcome. These reasons can range from a serious medical problem in the mother that affects the baby to actual physical problems with the uterus or placenta. In some cases, the cause for pre-maturity cannot be determined.

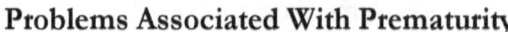

> **Problems Associated With Prematurity**
>
> *Lungs*
> Immature lungs are unable to properly perform their functions of providing oxygen and getting rid of carbon dioxide.
>
> *Eyes*
> Eyes are not completely developed. Scarring and vision loss can occur.
>
> *Digestive system*
> Immature suck and swallow along with under-developed intestines may require that the baby be fed through his veins.
>
> *Infection*
> Skin, which normally acts as a barrier to infection, is immature, allowing bacteria and other germs access to baby's system.

Post-maturity

Most people don't talk about babies being post-mature. When they do, it is usually to comment on how the mother must feel, as carrying a baby for any longer than expected can be a trial in and of itself!

The longer a baby is inside of the womb growing, the larger he can grow to be. Babies who

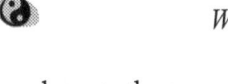

are larger than average can have trouble fitting through the vaginal canal. In addition, very large babies are sometimes unable to control their blood sugar levels in the period directly after birth.

Some post-mature infants will have the first bowel movement (called meconium) while still in the womb. This is noticed when the mother's water breaks and appears greenish-brown in color. A pediatrician specializing in newborn medicine (neonatologist) will be present at delivery to make sure that none of this stained fluid enters the baby's lungs.

Low Blood Sugar Levels

Low blood sugar levels in infants can occur for a variety of reasons. These include being larger or smaller than average, an infant of a diabetic mother, infection, prematurity and post-maturity. Whatever the reason, the outcomes of low blood sugar levels are what medical care providers try to avoid. When blood sugar levels drop too low, the baby can have seizures. Low blood sugar levels for too long can cause damage to the brain.

If you find that your baby is feeding poorly, seems unusually sleepy or just not acting right, you may want to ask to have blood his sugar level checked. This is a simple test that is done with a heel-stick to obtain a drop of blood, and the results are known in about 5 seconds.

Infection

Infection in a newborn infant is oftentimes difficult to detect. Some newborn babies (in fact, most) with serious infections will not get fevers. Instead, they may develop low body temperatures, begin to have trouble feeding, breathe more quickly, and just seem very sleepy.

Occasionally, the medical care provider has clues to be alert for infection: the mother is group B streptococcus positive or has known active herpes. In others, she must simply maintain a high index of suspicion to check for infection if a baby is not acting right.

To evaluate an infant for possible infection a blood sample is obtained. This sample is used to check a blood cell count and grow in the laboratory for possible bacteria and, if suspected, viruses. While waiting for the results, which can take up to 48 hours, most medical providers will provide antibiotic treatment to the baby through an IV. If all turns out well, the antibiotics are stopped. If the baby does have an infection, then the antibiotic choice is narrowed to be as specific as possible to the offending germ.

> If your baby is not acting right to you, say something! Parents are very in-tune with their children and are usually the first to notice a problem. Don't let anyone tell you that you're just being a "nervous mother."

Jaundice

Jaundice refers to the yellow tinge to the skin that can occur secondary to many different disease processes. Since the causes of jaundice vary, the treatment will depend on finding out the underlying problem.

Almost every newborn has a small amount of jaundice. This is referred to as "physiologic jaundice of the newborn." In order to understand where jaundice comes from, a review of the life of the red blood cell is in order.

Normal red blood cells in an adult have a lifespan of 120 days. At the end of their life cycle, these cells are recycled in a part of the body called the spleen. A protein called bilirubin is released into the bloodstream during this process. Bilirubin is broken down in the liver and eventually passed out of the body in bowel movements. It is the presence of high levels of bilirubin that gives skin a yellow color.

In a newborn infant, the average red blood cell lives only 90 days, so there is an increase in turnover of the products inside. While the baby is connected to his mother by the umbilical cord, the mother's body takes care of removing and breaking down bilirubin. However, once the baby is born, this connection is severed, and the baby now has to take over the management of bilirubin.

It takes a few days for the baby's liver to kick-in so, by about 3 or 5 days of age, the level of bilirubin can rise a little. This is mild, however, and does not cause damage. The baby will slowly resolve this himself.

In some instances, there is a problem in which the baby's red blood cells are destroyed at an even faster rate than usual. The bilirubin levels rise quickly and the baby becomes very yellow, usually within twenty-four hours of birth. One common cause of increased destruction of a baby's red blood cells is ABO incompatibility.

> "ABO" is the abbreviation for blood types: Type A, Type B, Type AB, and Type O. A mother who has Type O blood and carries a Type B or Type A infant will see her baby's red blood cells as "foreign" and make antibodies against them. These antibodies gain access to the baby by crossing over through the placenta, attack the baby's red blood cells and destroy them.

Very high levels of bilirubin can cause brain damage, so treatment is begun as soon as the rise in bilirubin begins to approach dangerous levels. Many people have seen babies under the blue lights in the nursery, wearing only a diaper and little eye-shields. The blue lights convert the bilirubin into a form that can be easily passed into the urine, thereby decreasing the amount in the blood.

Hospital Stay

During your baby's hospital stay he will be expected to do many things! Mostly, the medical staff will be observing him and taking note that all of his systems are working well. There will be some medications that are necessary to prevent possible disease, as well as tests to detect any disease he may have early enough to allow for treatment.

In the Delivery Room

Your baby's job at this point is simple: cry until he is not blue in the face! Babies are born with the little air sacs, or alveoli, of the lungs collapsed shut. In order to open them up, a baby will need to generate a breath about 4 times stronger than he will ever have to take again. No one will slap your baby on the bottom if he isn't crying, though. Back and foot rubbing are usually annoying enough to get the baby going.

Your baby will then be dried off and left under a warmer with a thermometer attached. The warmer provides enough heat to keep him at a stable body temperature. Once he is able to maintain this temperature on his own, he will be removed from under the warmer, wrapped snuggly in blankets and put in a little bassinette.

If your baby is doing well, there is no reason why you cannot hold him in the delivery room. If he is having a little trouble transitioning then he may need to spend a few hours in a special care nursery. But, you must be allowed to see him before he goes, even if for a brief second!

Eye Ointment and Vitamin K Injection

Shortly after your baby's delivery, he will receive two very important disease-preventing medications. These medications are given in what is called a "prophylactic" fashion. Waiting until the baby shows signs or symptoms of a problem before administering these medications would be too late.

Eye Ointment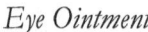

An antibiotic eye ointment is applied to the baby's eyes in order to prevent a serious eye-infection called conjunctivitis. This ointment is gooey and some medical-care providers advocate that the application be withheld until after the infant and his parents have had a chance to bond. They maintain that the presence of the ointment interferes with the infant's first visual contact with his parents. Speak with your medical care provider about your concerns in that regard.

Vitamin K Injection

Vitamin K prevents a serious bleeding problem that can occur in newborn infants. This vitamin is normally produced by bacteria that live in the intestines. Newborn infants do not have any bacteria in their intestines and, therefore, no source of vitamin K. The injection allows enough of this essential vitamin to be available for adequate blood clotting, until bacteria populate the baby's intestines and take over providing a supply of vitamin K.

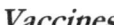

Vaccines

Within the first 24 to 48 hours after birth, most hospitals give newborn babies the hepatitis B vaccination. This is the first in a series of three injections and it is one of the few vaccinations that can actually prevent cancer (liver cancer, when caused by hepatitis B infection).

If you are infected with hepatitis B then your baby must receive this vaccine in the delivery room to aid in preventing transmission of the virus to his system. There is also an injection containing actual antibodies to hepatitis B that must be given to babies born to hepatitis B infected mothers.

> If you are hepatitis B positive, make sure that the necessary vaccines are present in the delivery room to allow for immediate administration.

Your Baby's First 24 Hours

The American Academy of Pediatrics recommends that babies be put to the breast as soon as possible within the first hour of life.[7] This is important for several reasons. First, it allows for the mother and her new baby to bond. Second, the baby will get his first "dose" of colostrum. Finally, stimulation of the mother's breasts will cause hormonal signals in her body to start production of milk. Mothers who have decided to bottle-feed should also feed their babies as soon as feasible to allow for bonding. In either case, early feeding can also help to prevent the baby's blood sugar level from falling too low.

Within the first few hours, your baby should be able to control his temperature. Babies who become cold-stressed are not able to shiver to generate heat yet. If your baby is having trouble keeping his temperature in the normal range after several hours, this is a sign that should not be ignored. Low body temperature can be a sign of serious infection!

All babies should pass urine within the first 24 hours. Failure to do so could be an indication of a problem somewhere along the urinary system.

> Many infants who are said to have not passed urine may have actually done so in the delivery room and it was either not observed or not documented.

Many hospitals now offer, and support, rooming-in, which is to say that the baby will actually stay with you in your room and not in a separate nursery. This type of rooming arrangement can be very helpful for a breastfeeding infant who will tend to want to feed more frequently.

Be aware that you can leave your baby in the nursery for a stretch if you need a chance for sleep. Take advantage of this time to rest! Once you get home, the demands will be great, and you just went through childbirth. Your body needs to recuperate. Do not feel guilty for wanting to sleep while your baby is temporarily cared for by the nurses.

The Next 24 Hours

If you had an uncomplicated vaginal delivery, you will most likely be allowed to go home 48 hours after your baby's birth. Some experienced mothers prefer to go home sooner, and, if all is well, may get the green light to do so.

By the end of the first 48 hours, your infant should have had his first bowel movement.

This first bowel movement consists of a thick, tarry substance called meconium. The first several bowel movements will be of this consistency, gradually changing in appearance over a period of a few days. Breast-fed infants usually have bowel movements that are mustard-yellow in color with what appear to be little seeds mixed in. Formula-fed infants tend to have stools that are more formed and darker in color.

Before your baby is discharged to go home with you, a test called a newborn screen is done. This test is usually obtained by pricking the baby's heel, obtaining drops of blood on a filter paper and then sending the sample off to a lab for analysis. The purpose of this screening is to allow for the identification of babies with disorders that can be treated when detected early, before complications arise. If any of the test results are abnormal, the state or other agency will contact you for further testing.

> Diseases included in the newborn screen vary by state and can include sickle-cell disease, hypothyroidism, certain defects in metabolism, and other genetic disorders.

Finally, many states have instituted mandatory newborn hearing tests on all infants before they are discharged from the hospital nursery. Most hearing disorders are not picked up until, on average, 2 years of age.[19] By identifying children with hearing loss earlier, important interventions can take place to give the child a better chance at communicating.

Going Home

When the day arrives for your hospital discharge, it can be a time of both excitement and fear. If this is your first baby, you may worry about suddenly being without the help of the nursing and support-staff of the hospital. You will suddenly be "flying solo." If there are other children at home, you may be wondering how they will take it when you have to dedicate so much time and attention to this new little person.

The hospital will most likely require that they see your baby properly secured in his car seat before they will let you leave. That first car seat installation can be quite frustrating, so you may want to figure out how to use it before the time comes to actually put the baby in it. Remember that you need to buckle up as well. Take the same care of yourself while riding in a vehicle as you do your precious infant.

The First Few Weeks

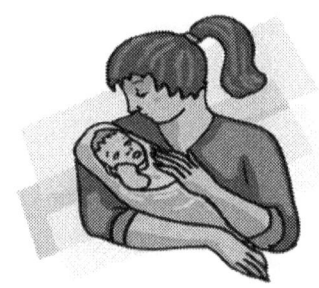

Now that you are at home with your new baby, you can begin to get to know each other in your natural setting, out of the hospital and away from some of the artificial schedules that can be imposed.

Although many people will want to visit, try to limit the traffic in and out of your home.

From Me To You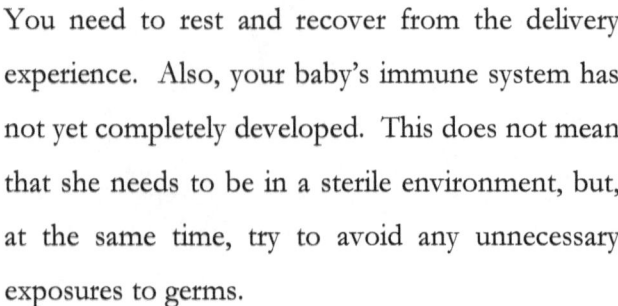

You need to rest and recover from the delivery experience. Also, your baby's immune system has not yet completely developed. This does not mean that she needs to be in a sterile environment, but, at the same time, try to avoid any unnecessary exposures to germs.

Day-to-Day Care
Feeding

There are different schools of thought regarding a child's feeding schedule. One asserts that a child needs to be placed on a feeding schedule from day one. The other counters by saying that a child should regulate her own schedule as she knows her needs best.

I tend to agree with the recommendation that an infant be allowed to assert her own needs. When a feeding schedule is forced upon a child, she will not be able to respond to her internal signals of hunger and fullness. While this may not seem to be a big issue, it can become one later. A recent study has shown that the more a mother (fathers were not included in this study) controls the feeding situation, the more likely a child is to develop later feeding problems.[20]

What does this mean for you? When your baby cries, feel free to offer her the breast (or bottle) in addition to determining whether there is another reason for her discomfort. If she feeds for ten minutes on one occasion and then forty-five minutes the next, it is okay. A breastfeeding infant will stop feeding when she feels satisfied. You cannot really gauge how many ounces she has taken in, so you will have to observe her behavioral cues (falling asleep, letting go of the nipple) to determine fullness. With bottle fed infants, there is sometimes a tendency to expect the child to finish an entire bottle. If you prepare 3 ounces and she drinks just one ounce, don't force more!

> The number of diapers that your baby wets and soils over a twenty-four hours period is a good indicator of her intake. If you are changing at least five wet and 3 to four soiled diapers per day then she is probably getting enough to eat.[61]

Sleeping

One of the more difficult aspects of caring for a newborn is the sleeping (or lack-thereof) schedule. People often say that a child has her "days and nights mixed-up." The baby will sleep all day, waking briefly to feed and go back to sleep, only to be awake at night every 2 hours (or less)! Part of the explanation for this may be that when your baby was still inside of you, she was lulled to sleep by your daily movements. However, in the evening as you slept, the absence of these movements allowed your baby to stay awake.

What can you do about this? Well, start with knowing that "this too shall pass." Next, try to develop an evening routine in order to help your baby become accustomed to the idea of night for sleep, day for play. Once your baby has been laid down to sleep, try to minimize any loud noises. This does not mean that the house must remain completely quiet; your infant needs to be able to sleep with the normal background noise of the family. This is just not the time to be putting the television on full blast or shouting.

When your baby does awaken during the night, do what needs to be done quickly and quietly. A nightlight can be very helpful to allow you to see your baby without turning on all the lights and awakening her completely. While feeding or changing your baby, try not to stimulate her too much with talking and playing. It may be fun for the first few months, but she will learn quickly that it is okay to get up at night and play, and that can be difficult to undo!

Try your best to stimulate your baby after each daytime feeding. This is not as easy as it sounds, as she will probably drift off to sleep during or immediately after her meal. With time, she will have longer and longer periods of alertness, which will give you more time to interact with her.

> ALWAYS place your baby on her back to sleep. Stomach sleeping has been associated with an increased risk of Sudden Infant Death Syndrome (SIDS).

One extremely important piece of advice, for your own sanity, is this: nap when your baby naps! There is always going to be that feeling inside that you should "get something done" while the baby is sleeping. Use your support system to help with things that must get done (laundry, dishes, meals). For other, less necessary chores, lower your standards for just a little while. Your home does not have to be in perfect order, just healthy and safe!

Another piece of advice regarding your infant's sleep is to have her sleep in your room with you. The controversy surrounding co-sleeping, which is broadly defined as either having the baby in the same room or same bed as you, continues. A middle-ground approach would be to have your baby sleeping directly along-side your bed in a bassinette or co-sleeper that attaches to, but is separate from, your bed

> By having your baby nearby, you can attend to her needs before she completely awakens. Once your child is screaming, it may take a while to calm her back down in order to feed her.

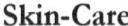

Skin-Care

It will take several weeks for your baby to develop the smooth, silky skin that babies are known for. Immediately after birth, you may have noticed that your baby was covered with a thick, white, cheesy substance. This substance is called "vernix caseosa" and is composed of accumulated skin cells that the baby has shed while developing in your womb. Vernix caseosa serves as a protective barrier during the time that your baby was immersed 24/7 in your amniotic fluid.

Once the vernix caseosa is removed, the baby's skin may become dry and peel, especially in the areas around the wrists and ankles. If this peeling becomes severe and cracks, speak with your child's medical provider. Otherwise, the dryness will slowly resolve as her skin begins to produce its own natural oils.

> Be careful if you decide to apply lotion to your infant's skin. Some of the perfumes in lotions and creams, even those formulated for babies, may cause irritation.

While your baby's umbilical cord is still in place and the area is healing, it is best to sponge-bathe her. You want to keep the cord area as dry as possible, so that it can fall off more quickly. Do not be afraid to gently lift the cord up and down in order to apply alcohol to the area directly beneath that is still moist and yellow. This will not hurt your baby! She may cry at the feel of the cool alcohol on her skin.

Do not use a cotton-swab or other blunt object to apply alcohol to the umbilical cord. Just dip a cotton ball into the alcohol, and then gently dab it around the cord site. You may notice a yellowish discharge from the cord-site, which is not a sign of infection. A small amount of this fluid is normal.

> If there is a large amount of yellow-green or blood-tinged fluid from the cord site associated with an abnormal smell and swelling or redness around the belly button, have your child examined by her healthcare provider at once.

After the umbilical cord falls off, there may still be a small area of healing just inside of the belly button. You do not need to pry this area open in order to apply alcohol; it will heal with time. It is now okay to bathe your baby. Have your camera ready to capture this important first!

Hair Care

When a baby is born she may be bald, have a full head of hair or anything in-between. The first hair of a baby is usually very fine in texture and gradually lost over the first four months of life. This hair will be replaced by hair that may be of a different texture and/or color.[22]

Scientists have categorized hair types into three general categories in their purest forms: Asian, Caucasoid and.[39] All hair is composed of a protein called keratin which is arranged in bundles to form the hair shaft. In Asian hair, the shaft is almost completely round with straight keratin bundles. Caucasoid hair has mixed proportions of straight and wavy keratin bundles with oval-shaped shafts. This accounts for the large variety of hair textures in this type. Finally, pure African hair has wavy keratin bundles with many twists in the shaft, which leads to its ultra-curled appearance. The shaft is oval but the edges are "kinked" subjecting them to damage.

Due to the genetically mixed nature of many African-Americans, our hair tends to not be of the pure African type. Most of us do have texture to our hair, however, and the underlying structure makes it more susceptible to damage. When caring for your baby's hair, handle it gently. Excessive pulling and tugging can break the shaft. After washing the hair, you may want to apply a light oil preparation to maintain softness of the curl pattern.

Finally, when arranging your baby's hair into a style, be careful with how tightly you pull it. Securing the hair tightly with barrettes or tightly braiding it will cause hair loss.

Taking Care of Yourself

You are allowed to be tired, to want a break, to have some "me" time, and to be sure that you get it! By taking care of yourself, you will be better for you and your family. This time for

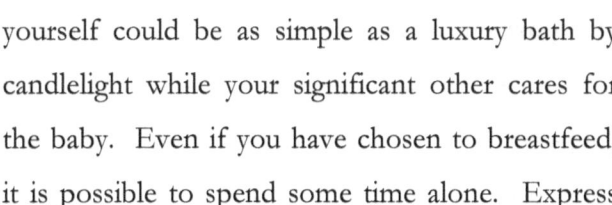

yourself could be as simple as a luxury bath by candlelight while your significant other cares for the baby. Even if you have chosen to breastfeed, it is possible to spend some time alone. Express some milk and go take a breather.

Postpartum Check

Remember to keep your postpartum follow-up appointment with your obstetrical provider. The timing of this visit can vary from two weeks to six weeks after delivery, depending on the type of delivery. Even if you feel "fine," this check-up is necessary to assure that you are healing well. It is also a time to discuss reliable contraceptive methods. In addition, it may be time for your yearly PAP examination.

Many women put themselves last on the list and when time gets tight, their own needs are the first to be put off. Plan in advance on how you will get to your appointment, and just go!

> You can become pregnant even if you are breastfeeding and have not yet resumed menstruation.

From Me To You

Postpartum Depression

Media images portray that a new mother is supposed to be happy and elated with the entire process of her pregnancy, delivery and new baby. This stereotype leaves many new mothers questioning why they feel less than happy at times after bringing their baby home. These feelings, termed the baby blues, are normal. They are experienced by up to 80 percent of new mothers.[32]

Affected women will notice that they are more tearful than usual, with mood swings between happiness and sadness and some difficulty concentrating. These normal occurrences are due to the rapid shift in hormone levels that occurs both immediately and for a few weeks after birth. Baby blues usually occur within the first week after birth and tend to subside after a two-week period.

Of major concern is postpartum depression, a condition that affects 15-20% of new mothers.[32] The symptoms usually appear gradually but can occur rapidly and can begin any time during the first year! Women with postpartum depression feel extreme fatigue, suffer from excess worrying, changes in appetite with either significant weight loss or gain, and a lack of feeling towards the baby.

Women who have a prior history of postpartum depression have a 50 to 80 percent increased risk of developing postpartum depression after later pregnancies.[32] Furthermore, women with a history of depression prior to pregnancy, as well as those without support systems, have more likelihood of developing this disorder.

If you are concerned that you have or are developing postpartum depression, get help! Speak with your obstetrical provider or a trusted friend or family member. By not seeking treatment, you will create unnecessary suffering for yourself and your family. Research has shown that children in homes with mothers who are not treated for depression are more likely to have psychiatric issues themselves, as well as later behavioral and learning problems.[32] If you are having trouble finding help, please see Appendix A for postpartum depression support web links.

The First Year

Your Baby's First Year of Check-Ups

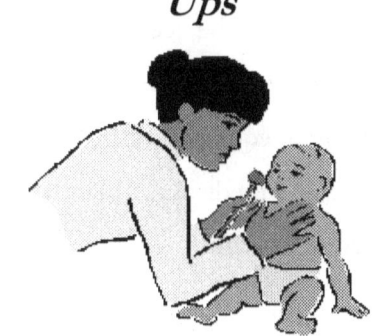

The current guidelines for healthcare exams (also called well-baby exams) set forth by the American Academy of Pediatrics are as follows:

- Within two weeks of birth
- 2 months
- 4 months
- 6 months
- 9 months
- 12 months

It is imperative that your baby be examined at these intervals, even if he seems healthy. At these visits, measurements are made to ensure that your child is growing adequately. Oftentimes, the only clue that there is a medical problem is a shift in a child's pattern of growth.

> At well-baby visits, your baby's development will be assessed, vaccinations administered and screening tests done, all with the purpose of identifying problems before they arise.

Your Baby's First Year Of Check-Ups

The well-baby visits are perfect times for parents to speak with their child's healthcare provider regarding any concerns. These visits can also serve as opportunities to receive anticipatory guidance, or what to expect in the coming months. I suggest that you write down any questions that you may have before the visit, as once in the exam room, it is easy to forget all that you wanted to ask

This chapter contains areas in which you can record your baby's measurements at each medical office visit. There is also space to jot down any questions that you may have and all advice that was given to you by your child's healthcare provider. There is even a spot to place a picture of your baby at each interval. You will be amazed upon looking back at these photos how much your baby will have changed in just one year's time!

From Me To You

My Baby's First Visit

Date:

My questions for this visit:

Weight: Length: Head:

Feeding:

Immunizations:

Advice given:

Next visit:

Newborn Visit

Most medical providers prefer to see a newborn infant within two weeks of hospital discharge or sooner if there were problems at the time of delivery or during the hospital stay. Ideally, the baby's healthcare provider would examine him in the hospital; however, many medical practices utilize the hospital's in-house pediatricians for the care of newborn infants.

> Make sure that you bring any hospital papers to the first well baby exam. These will have your baby's delivery history, measurements, hepatitis B vaccination date, and hearing screen results.

General

At the newborn visit, your baby will receive a head-to-toe examination. He will be weighed, and his length and head circumference measured. These measurements will then be plotted on a growth chart, which will compare his growth to the growth of other infants his age.

It is normal for a healthy newborn infant to lose up to 10% of his birth-weight in the first few days after birth; however, this weight should be regained, and the baby back to birth-weight, by the 10th day of life.

> Growth charts are based on the normal growth patterns of infants who have been fed infant formula. The growth of breastfed infants is different, and this should be taken into consideration when interpreting the charts.

Development

While examining the different systems of your baby's body, the healthcare-provider is making an overall assessment of your child in terms of how he moves and responds to stimuli. Newborn babies tend to hold their arms and legs in a flexed position, bent at the elbows and knees. There are also several normal reflexes that should be present. Their presence helps to confirm that the nervous system is intact and functioning.

Newborn Reflexes

Grasp

A newborn should grasp anything that is placed into his palm. This same response should occur with the soles of his feet.

Startle

Officially known as the Moro reflex, this one occurs when the baby is suddenly laid flat on his back. The arms shoot out to the side, then back in, and he cries.

Rooting

Baby will turn his face to the side and open his mouth when his cheek is stroked. This reflex can be useful when trying to get the baby to open his mouth wide to breastfeed.

Vaccines

If your baby did not receive his first hepatitis B vaccine in the hospital then it will be given today.

Feeding

Your baby's medical care provider will speak with you regarding the baby's feeding patterns. If you are breastfeeding, this is an excellent opportunity to review any Common Concerns that sometimes arise early on. These include pain from engorgement, latch-on difficulties and sore nipples. If your baby's provider is not comfortable answering these questions, request a referral to someone who can (such as a lactation consultant or visiting nurse).

Common Concerns

ଔ *Acrocyanosis*

A common finding in newborns that causes parental concern is acrocyanosis, or bluish-purple hands and feet. The discoloration is due to poor blood circulation to the hands and feet. The blood vessels serving those areas in newborns are very

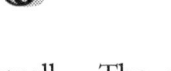

small. The color change is most pronounced when the baby is cold and the blood vessels constrict to conserve heat. This will resolve as the baby grows.

❧ Hiccups

Many babies will have hiccups, which is nothing more than a reflex of the diaphragm, the primary muscle used for breathing. Do not give your baby water to make the hiccups stop. This does not work, and can actually be dangerous in an infant this age.

❧ *Umbilical cord discharge*

Another common occurrence is a mild discharge from the umbilical cord site. This occurs as the area is healing, and its presence is not a sign of infection. However, if the site becomes red, or there is a large amount of foul-smelling discharge, you should have your baby checked-out.

What to Watch Out For

Finally, your provider will go over some warning signs that there may be a problem. An infant this age showing any of these signs should be taken for immediate medical attention.

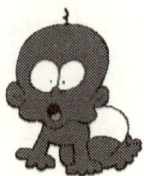

- ~ Fever (higher than 100.4 F rectal) OR low temperature
- ~ Poor feeding/difficult to arouse
- ~ Excessive vomiting, or green-tinged vomit

No water

A baby's kidneys are not yet mature enough to handle water. When water levels become too high in the blood, the baby could have seizures and permanent brain damage.

Never shake a baby

Shaking a baby, even if just for a second, can cause "shaken baby syndrome," which has permanent, life-long effects and can even cause death.

No honey

Honey contains small amounts of a toxin called botulinum. The amount present does not cause problems in adults or older children, but, in infants under one year of age, can cause paralysis and death.

Your Baby's First Year Of Check-Ups

2 Months Old!

Date:

My questions for this visit:

Weight: Length: Head:

Feeding:

Immunizations:

Advice given:

Next visit:

2 Month Visit

Your baby's measurements will be taken again, and you should discuss with your doctor any problems or concerns that have arisen since the last visit. In particular, please be sure to let your provider know of any visits to the emergency room or hospitalizations.

Development

The development of a two month old reflects the fact that muscular control proceeds from the neck down. By this age, the baby should be able to hold his head steady and to lift his head up if placed down on his stomach. Remember, though, to ALWAYS lay your baby down on his back to sleep, unless otherwise directed by your medical provider.

You will also notice that your baby begins to coo and smile. You may get your first "responsive smile", which is when the baby is actually smiling in response to seeing you! When your baby coos, talk back. This is how he learns language as well as social skills. Do not be afraid to speak normally. Many people speak baby talk to an infant, but the more you talk to your baby in adult language, the more he will learn. Of course, have some fun too, and imitate some of the sounds that your baby has made. This will show him that you are listening, and you do hear him!

Vaccines

This is the visit that many new parents dread. It is at this visit that the first vaccines to protect against diptheria, pertussis, haemophilus influenza type b, tetanus, polio, rotavirus and pneumococcus are given. Fortunately, there are several combination vaccines available on the market that can decrease the number of injections that your child has to receive. As an added plus, the rotavirus vaccine is in liquid form that is given through your baby's mouth.

The vaccines and recommended ages for administration outlined below are only guidelines. Depending on the manufacturer and type of combination vaccination used, your child's individual schedule may differ.

Vaccine	Disease(s) Prevented	Age
DTaP	Diptheria, Tetanus and Pertussis	2, 4, 6 months
Hib	Haemophilus type B bacterial meningitis	2, 4, 6 months
IPV	Polio	2, 4, 6, months
Prevnar	Pneumococcal meningitis	2, 4, 6, 12 months
Hepatitis B	Hepatitis B infection	Birth, 2, and 6 months
Rotavirus	Viral gastroenteritis	2, 4, 6 months
MMR	Measles, Mumps and Rubella	12 months
Varivax	Varicella (Chickenpox)	12 months
Hepatitis A	Hepatitis A infection	12 months

A Brief History of Vaccination[37]

Edward Jenner, MD, was an English surgeon. In May of the year 1796, Dr. Jenner noticed that milkmaids who had been infected with cowpox were immune to smallpox. He took a cowpox-infected skin sample from a milkmaid named Sarah Nelmes and injected it into an eight year old boy named James Phipp. The little boy had a mild illness for about 10 days, and then completely recovered. Dr. Jenner then **injected the boy with smallpox** and the child did not develop the disease! This technique was then copied and repeated to create the smallpox vaccine.

The word vaccine comes from the Latin word "vacca" which means cow; this is a direct result of the origin of the first commonly used vaccines.

Common vaccine concerns

In response to much of the recent media attention given to vaccines, their components and even their necessity, the Centers for Disease Control and Prevention has issued several reviews of the current perceptions present in many parents' minds in this regard.

The CDC discusses six common beliefs held by parents who may choose to withhold vaccines from their children in the article "Six Common Misconceptions About Vaccination, and How to Respond to Them."[27] The beliefs include:

> "Diseases had already begun to disappear before vaccines were introduced, because of better hygiene and sanitation"

> "The majority of people who get a disease have been vaccinated"

> "There are 'hot lots' of vaccines that have been associated with more adverse events and deaths than others"

"Vaccines cause many harmful side effects, illnesses, and even death"

"Vaccine-preventable diseases have been virtually eliminated from the United States"

"Giving a child multiple vaccinations for different diseases at the same time increases the risk of harmful side effects and can overload the immune system"

The bottom line is that extensive research has been done on the safety and efficacy of each vaccine before it is recommended for general use. There is also an "adverse reaction reporting system," in which any reaction to a vaccine is immediately reported to determine if there is a reason for concern. This means that there is ongoing surveillance for vaccine reactions in order to assure the public that the vaccines they are receiving are safe.

In a second article entitled "What Would Happen if We Stopped Vaccinations,"[28] the CDC points out the devastating consequences of eliminating the practice of vaccination with the assumption that the diseases we vaccinate against are no longer in existence.

They recount the history of the haemophilus influenzae type b (Hib) vaccine that was developed and introduced for routine use in 1987. Before that time, one in every 200 children living in the United States of America became ill from Hib, with severe illnesses such as meningitis, blood infections and pneumonia. In particular, 600 children per year were killed by Hib-caused meningitis and many children who did survive had long-term after-effects such as deafness, seizure disorders and mental retardation.

Since the routine use of the Hib vaccine, the incidence of Hib infections has dropped by 98%, with less than 10 fatal cases in a ten-year period! If this vaccine were discontinued, there would be a quick return to the disease rates seen in the 1980's.[28]

Hib vaccination is just one example of many. Due to the global nature of travel, there is a continuous threat of exposure to certain infectious agents that, if not immunized against, can cause severe illness in children. In one case in California, there was a diphtheria exposure in a school; the only child who died was the one who was not vaccinated.[28]

Feeding

Breast milk or formula is still all that your baby needs. All parents have a relative who tells them "that baby needs some food." At the baby's first whimper or suck on the hand, this person interprets hunger. Remember, not all sucking indicates hunger. Babies use sucking to soothe and calm themselves. Some infants will take to pacifiers, others, their hands and still others, their mother's nipple! Not all cries mean hunger either. Investigate the other common reasons for crying if it has not been awhile since your child was last fed. Does he have a wet or soiled diaper? Is he hot, tired or over-stimulated?

It is not recommended to start solid foods until the age of 6 months. Until that time, your baby gets all of the calories that he needs to grow from breast milk or formula. Starting solid food sooner could actually be dangerous. Your baby's neuromuscular development is not yet complete in the neck and chest, making coordination of swallowing food difficult. This could put your baby at increased risk for choking

> Children who start solid foods earlier may develop more food allergies.[21] They may also take in too many calories, especially if the food is mixed in with milk in a bottle.

And, what about the age-old advice about giving the baby a cereal bottle, to help him sleep through the night? As a parent who has tried this herself, I can tell you that it does not work. I still had many sleepless nights, which is part of having an infant at home!

If your baby is exclusively breastfed or receives less than 16 ounces of vitamin D fortified infant formula per day, then he needs to begin supplemental vitamin D drops at this time.[23] Vitamin D is essential for the production of strong, healthy bones. Although there is some vitamin D present in breast milk, it may not be in a sufficient quantity to support bone growth.

Vitamin D is produced by the body in the skin. This reaction requires sunlight. Darker-skinned individuals need more sunlight exposure to produce the same amount of vitamin D as lighter-skinned persons.[23] For that reason, darker-skinned babies who are exclusively breast-fed by darker-skinned mothers run the highest risk of having vitamin D deficiency. This could further lead to soft bones and the development of the disease rickets.

> Rickets is characterized by bones that are so soft that they bend, leading to bowed-legs, wide wrists and even abnormally shaped ribs.

From Me To You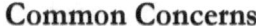

Common Concerns

ଓଃ *Bowel movements*

Many infants at this age will begin to experience a change in the pattern of their bowel movements. In the first few months of life, your infant may have had a bowel movement during or immediately after each feeding. However, now that his bowels are maturing, the reflex to immediately have a bowel movement is decreasing and he may have dramatically fewer movements over the course of the day. This is not a sign of constipation, especially if the stools are soft. The baby may appear to be straining or using a lot of force to pass his bowel movements, but this is only because he has to use all of his strength to push (imagine if you tried to have a bowel movement on your back)!

What to Watch Out For

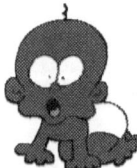

Even if you think that your baby cannot roll over, NEVER leave him unattended on a high surface (such as a bed, couch or changing table).

Your Baby's First Year Of Check-Ups

4 Months Old!

Date:

My questions for this visit:

Weight: Length: Head:

Feeding:

Immunizations:

Advice given:

Next visit:

From Me To You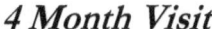

4 Month Visit

This well-baby visit will be very much like the last. Fortunately, babies are generally healthy, and their main job is to grow! As such, even if your baby seems well, he still needs to have his scheduled check-ups. If there is a problem with his growth (weight, length, or head measurements), it may be a sign of an underlying problem.

As always, inform your healthcare provider of any serious illnesses or emergency room visits that may have occurred since your baby's last check-up.

Development

Your baby will be observed by the healthcare provider very closely to ascertain his developmental stage. While it may not be obvious to you, the provider is watching how your baby moves, how he interacts with you and how he responds to different stimuli. This will give an idea of whether or not your baby is on-track with his developmental milestones.

All babies develop at their own paces, and there is a range of normal. But, if your child's development appears to be delayed in any way, it is better to address it early with a formal evaluation by a developmental specialist. Many states have programs called "Early-Intervention Programs" whose very existence is to provide services to children when they are younger and will benefit most from treatments. The "watch-and-wait" method is a disservice to any child who may be developing more slowly than normal.

> Nerve connections and brain growth are still occurring in your growing baby; the earlier that an intervention is put into effect (e.g. physical therapy), the more benefits your child will reap.

You can expect your baby to do some or all of the following at this age:

- Look at his own hand
- Bring both hands together in front of his face
- Turn towards a sound

- Bear weight on his legs (this will not cause your child to become bow-legged, contrary to popular belief)
- Coo/babble

Vaccines

As of the date of the print of this book, the following vaccines are recommended at age 4 months: DTaP, Hib, IPV, prevnar, hepatitis B (if given as part of a combination vaccine) and rotavirus. Make your child's medical provider aware of any prior reactions to the first set of vaccines.

> Even if your baby is ill at the time of his well-baby check-up it may still be possible for him to be vaccinated. For a list of the absolute circumstances under which a vaccine should not be given, visit the Centers for Disease Control's website (See Appendix A).

Feeding

Remember, breast milk or formula is **still** all that your baby needs at this time. More and more, people around you may pressure you to begin to feed your baby cereal, fruit, juice, or water. Try to resist this pressure. Your baby is growing at the fastest rate that he ever will in his life; he needs to receive all of the calories and balanced nutrients available in breast milk or formula for optimal growth. Point out to these well-meaning advisers that your baby is growing well, and that you will be waiting until he is six months old before introducing solids.

Common Concerns

༄ *Spoiling*

Many parents worry that they will spoil their child by "giving in" too easily. Some believe that a baby should not be held often or that his cries need not be immediately answered. The fear is that the child will grow to become demanding, defiant and difficult to handle.

At four months of age, there is no chance of spoiling your child by responding to his cries or holding and hugging him. These early months of his life are the foundation for the rest of his days. He is learning about human interaction and, above all else, trust. There has been much attention and research put into the importance of early attachment and its necessity to be able to form relationships and be successful later in life.

The so-called "attachment bond" develops after birth, when an infant's needs are met in a consistent and loving manner by a consistently present primary caretaker. These experiences are absolutely necessary for continued normal development of an infant's brain. Certain nerve connections are still being made and brain growth occurring. In severe cases of emotional neglect children's brains will actually stop growing![52]

Children with secure attachment bonds do better overall in "forming friendships, relationships with teachers, coaches, siblings, and, over time, in the workplace and larger community."[52] Our African-American culture has tended to warn against holding babies too much, and, especially in our boys, we don't want to be too soft on them.

Give your baby the best emotional base that you can by holding and loving him and responding to his needs consistently. Turn a deaf ear to those who say that you are spoiling him.

What to Watch Out For

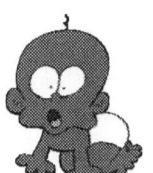

> By 4 months of age, most infants are bringing their hands, and anything in them, to their mouths. The risk of choking is greatly increased, so never leave small objects within your baby's reach.

From Me To You

6 Months Old!

Date:

My questions for this visit:

Weight:		Length:		Head:

Feeding:

Immunizations:

Advice given:

Next visit:

6 Month Visit

As before, your baby will be weighed and his head and length will be measured. Notify your physician of any illness or emergency room visits/hospitalizations that your child may have had.

Development

Your baby's nervous system development has continued down past his head, neck and chest, and is moving downward towards his lower trunk and torso. As such, he will begin to gain control over his lower back and hip muscles, all of which will be reflected in the new things he will start to do!

He will also be experimenting with noises and sounds. You may find that upon discovering how to make a new sound, your baby will repeat it over and over for several days before moving on to the next one. These sounds include gurgling, squeals and, sometimes, even coughs!

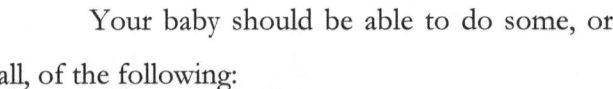

Your baby should be able to do some, or all, of the following:

- ~ Feed himself
- ~ Pass a toy from hand to hand
- ~ Say "Dada" or "Mama", but not specifically (does not use the words specifically for his mother or father)
- ~ Roll over

Feeding

NOW is the time to begin feeding your baby what are called "complementary foods." These feedings are called complementary because they are meant to only complement bottle or breast-feeding, not replace them.

> Your infant will still receive most of his nutrition from breast milk or formula. The introduction of other forms of feeding can and should occur over the process of several months.

It is usually very easy to tell that your baby is ready to start trying out cereals, fruits and veggies. Physically, he should have good support of the upper body, an indirect sign that his muscular development is adequate for the eating process (chewing, swallowing). Socially, you will notice that he has an interest in food when you are eating; he reaches for your plate, and watches intently as you lift each forkful to your mouth!

Remember, start your baby off slowly. Do not expect him to automatically take to the spoon and eagerly open his mouth for each serving. It is recommended that you begin with a single-ingredient food such as infant rice cereal. These cereals are available commercially and are iron-fortified. The incidence of allergy to rice cereal is very low, making it an ideal starter-food.

Begin by mixing a very small amount of cereal in a bowl (NOT THE BOTTLE) with some breast milk or formula. It should be of a slightly runny consistency. Hold the spoon to the baby's lips and let him suck the cereal off. He may use his tongue to push some of the food back out and make some faces of disgust, but this is just because he is trying something new. After a few spoonfuls, stop for that feeding. Gradually increase the amount of each feeding, as well as the consistency of the cereal.

After about two weeks, when your baby is accustomed to the spoon and does well with the rice cereal, you can begin to introduce other foods. Some parents will offer oatmeal, barley or other single-grain infant cereal next. You can also try fruits and vegetables. The order in which you introduce them is not important.

Allow for at least three days to pass between the introduction of each new food (ideally, five days to a week), in order that you can identify any possible allergic reactions. It is also for this reason that single ingredient foods are to be used. Giving mixed-ingredient foods at this stage can cause confusion if an allergic reaction occurs; you will not know which component of the food your infant had the reaction to.

The following two in-sets include information on foods to avoid during the first year, as well as information on making your own baby food.

Foods to Avoid in the First Year

Make sure that those who provide any childcare for your baby are aware of the foods that are not to be given to your child.

Choking Hazards

Hot dogs (cut into round pieces)
Raw carrots or hard fresh fruits (in whole or large pieces)
Fruits with pits
Grapes
Peanut butter
Nuts

Risk of Allergy/Irritation

Egg whites
Peanuts
Soy
Dairy products
Citrus

Making Your Own Baby Food

An entire market has evolved around the feeding of infants and children. It is easy to become accustomed to the convenience of jarred baby food and begin to rely on it. Making food yourself assures that it is fresh and you will know exactly what ingredients are present. Your baby will become accustomed to real foods and not those that are prepackaged, setting the foundation for healthier eating habits later in life.

There are several books available on the subject along with interesting recipes that your baby is sure to enjoy. One personal favorite of mine is Baby Blender Food. This book gives wonderful tips on safe preparation and storage of foods for your baby (see Appendix A).

Vaccines

The current recommendations for this age group are: DTaP, Hib, IPV, prevnar, hepatitis B, and rotavirus. If you are currently in the winter season, your baby should receive the flu vaccine as well.

Common Concerns

○8 *Crawling*

Many parents will ask me "when will my baby start to crawl?" Interestingly, the acquisition of this skill is not even included in routine developmental assessments. Some children actually skip this milestone, as they may find that they can get from place to place by rolling or commando crawling (pulling themselves forward with their arms while lying flat on their bellies).

Even fewer infants may be crawling these days as a consequence of the "Back-to-Sleep" campaign to help prevent SIDS (sudden infant death syndrome). Infants and babies are spending less time on their stomachs and, thus, using those skills less often. If you want to encourage your baby's development, give him plenty of "tummy time" when he is awake. At that time, he can explore the

From Me To You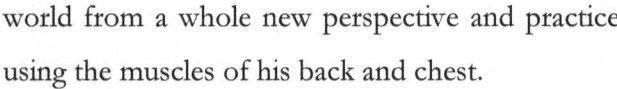

world from a whole new perspective and practice using the muscles of his back and chest.

What to Watch Out For

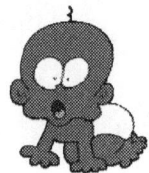

If it appears to you that your baby has trouble hearing, have him evaluated, EVEN IF he passed his newborn hearing test. Some hearing problems come later in life and parents are usually the first to pick up on it.

Your Baby's First Year Of Check-Ups

9 Months Old!

Date:

My questions for this visit:

Weight:　　　Length:　　　Head:

Feeding:

Immunizations:

Advice given:

Next visit:

9 Month Visit

The same routine applies at this visit as in all others. Your baby will be weighed and measured and you will speak with his medical care provider regarding any illnesses or hospital visits since the last check-up.

Some providers will also check for anemia and a blood lead level at this age. If blood tests will be done, request that a test for G6PD deficiency be sent. G6PD deficency is a red blood cell enzyme deficiency that is more common in African-Americans. If your baby was not tested for sickle-cell trait as part of his newborn screen, ask for this test as well.

Development

It may appear to you at this stage in your child's life that he does something new everyday! One of the more exciting milestones is when your baby pulls up on the edge of an object and stands. Once your child has mastered this skill, he will begin to do what we call cruising, in which he circles around objects while holding on.

The developmental milestones at this age include:

~ Saying "Mama" or "Dada" specifically to Mom or Dad
~ Waving "Bye-bye"
~ Indicating wants (usually by screaming or grunting)
~ Picking up objects with a precise thumb-finger grasp

Vaccines

There are usually no vaccines recommended at this age; however, if your child has missed any immunizations, or was truly ill when his last set was due, then they can be given today. If you are in the winter months, the flu vaccine should be given.

Feeding

Continue with the introduction of new foods to your infant, still avoiding the foods that can cause problems as outlined in the section on the sixth month of life. Also, you can give your baby combination foods, such as rice and chicken.

Just remember to make sure that he has had each ingredient previously as a single-ingredient food and had no reaction to it.

This is a wonderful time to introduce your baby to the use of a cup. "Sippy" cups are oftentimes used as a transition from bottle to cup. You can give your child water, breast milk or formula in the cup. Do not let him carry the cup around all day and take sips from it at-will. Drinking from a cup for long intervals of time will allow for an almost constant bathing of the teeth with milk or other liquids and increases your baby's risk of developing cavities or "baby-bottle rot."

> Try to limit your baby's intake of juice to 4 to 6 ounces per day. Juice is high in sugar and the intake of large amounts can actually cause diarrhea.

Common Concerns

ଓଃ *Teething*

A baby's first tooth may appear at around 6 to 10 months of age.[18] These ages are averages, which means that some babies get teeth sooner (my first son got his first tooth on the day he turned three months old) or later (his cousin got hers at twelve months). If your baby does not have teeth yet, don't worry. He is still within the range of normal.

ଓଃ *Separation Anxiety*

Most children will begin to experience some distress when they are separated from their parents at this age.[44] As a newborn infant, your child had no real concept of objects existing around him. However, he quickly learns that you are a separate entity but does not realize that your being out of sight does not mean that you are gone for good!

If your baby attends daycare, you may notice that he now becomes clingy and screams when you leave for the day. Or, perhaps your baby was accustomed to lying down for bed at night and now screams and screams unless you are by his side.

You can help your baby through this stage by being consistent. When he must be left in the care of another individual, develop a goodbye routine, in which you give him a hug and kiss and then depart. Do not stretch out the goodbye, it only makes things worse. If you were to speak with most daycare providers, they would tell you that the crying usually stops shortly after the parent is out of site and the child is distracted by an interesting toy or friend!

What to Watch Out For

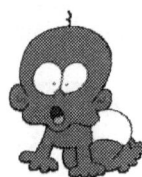

As your child becomes more mobile, increase your level of vigilance for objects that pose a threat to his safety. This includes household items that were previously out of reach by being placed on a coffee table, or cups of hot liquid that can be pulled off the edge of a table.

Your Baby's First Year Of Check-Ups

One Year Old!

Date:

My questions for this visit:

Weight: Length: Head:

Feeding:

Immunizations:

Advice given:

Next visit:

One year visit

Happy Birthday! One year ago, you had a newborn infant in your home who did little more than eat, sleep, cry, and poop. Now, just a short 12 months later, you have a dynamic, ever changing child who will never cease to amaze you with all that he learns! Each day will reveal something new about your child. This is a wonderful time period of life for both parents and children.

As always, when you take your child for his check-up, the medical care provider will measure him, in order to assure that he is growing well. Also, if it was not done at the 9 month-old visit, your baby will be checked for elevated blood lead levels and anemia. Remember to request the tests for G6PD deficiency and sickle-cell trait.

Development

Most one year olds have at least one word other than Mama or Dada that they say consistently. The more you talk to your child, the more his language will grow. He is a sponge absorbing all that occurs around him!

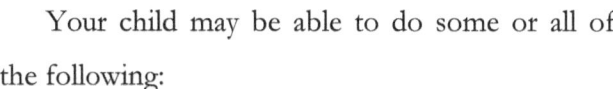
Your Baby's First Year Of Check-Ups

Your child may be able to do some or all of the following:

- Imitate activities (e.g. pretend to be talking on the telephone)
- Drink from a cup
- Stand alone
- Walk

Vaccines

The vaccines that are recommended at the 12-month visit as of the time of print of this book are: MMR (measles, mumps, and rubella), Varivax (chickenpox), prevnar, and hepatitis A.

Feeding

At this stage, your baby will probably be eating many different food combinations. If you have been formula feeding, now is the time to switch to whole cow's milk. Never give low-fat or nonfat milk to a child under the age of two years; Whole milk provides the necessary amount of fat to support your baby's rapidly developing nervous system.

If you are breastfeeding, there is no reason to stop just because your child has reached the one-year mark. The American Academy of Pediatrics recommends breastfeeding throughout a child's first year of life and then for as long thereafter as is preferred by the mother and child.[7] There will of course be people with the well meaning "you're still breastfeeding that baby?" Know that by continuing to breastfeed, you are also continuing to provide all of the known medical, social and emotional benefits that it carries.

Common Concerns

෬ *Not Walking*

Approximately 25% of all one year-olds walk well. That means 75% of them do not! The upper limit of normal for beginning to walk is 15 months of age. If your child is not yet walking, do not worry. As long as he has met all of his other milestones (pulling to stand, cruising around objects while holding on, standing alone), it will only be a matter of time before he starts walking.

❧ Bow-legged

One of the most Common Concerns that I have found exists among the African-American families that I provide pediatric care for is that their child seems "bow-legged." This refers to the curving outwards of the lower legs (the area below the knees).

In most cases, there is no problem and the legs will eventually reach a straighter appearance in a few years. The cases in which there should be concern include sudden appearance of bowed-legs or legs that are so bowed that they cause the child to fall frequently. In these instances, have your child evaluated to determine the underlying cause.

What to Watch Out For

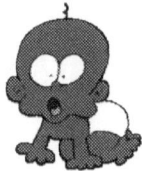

> Be especially careful to take good care of your baby's teeth. Many parents are not aware of the need to begin brushing their infant's teeth as soon as they appear. This will prevent cavities that can lead to tooth loss.

Common Occurrences During The First Year

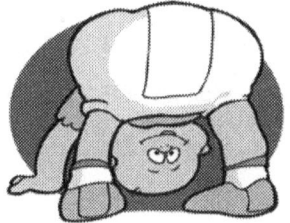

This section of the book will provide a systems-organized approach to many of the issues commonly encountered in the first year of a child's life. The review is not all-inclusive, nor does the inclusion of a particular topic mean that your child will encounter that situation. As with everything else, if you are at all concerned with your child's health or well being, have her evaluated by her medical care provider.

Head, Eyes, Ear, Nose, and Throat

During the first year of life, your baby will likely experience several upper respiratory infections, as well as an ear infection or two. The risk is even higher in those children in group daycare settings, as their exposure to germs is much higher than those at home. In addition to infections, there are several common conditions that affect the head, eyes, ears, nose, and throat, all of which are discussed below.

Head

Caput and Cephalohematoma

Despite their scary names, these are both more-or-less bruises of the scalp that can occur during a normal delivery. They give the head a "lop-sided" appearance but will resolve over time. Neither is related to brain injury and your pediatrician (and you) will just watch it disappear over the next few months.

Positional Molding

Some babies will develop flattening of the head on one side or, especially, the back of the head depending on how they are laying most of the time. Since the recommendation to lay babies down to sleep on their backs to reduce the risk of SIDS, many infants have developed this flattening along with some hair loss. When it was recommended that babies be placed on the side to sleep, flattening of one side of the face was seen. Rest assured that the head will regain its normal shape over time.

Eyes

Vision

For some time, people thought that infants are blind at birth. This belief still exists, as some of my patients will ask me at their baby's first check-up "when will she be able to see?"

In normally developed infants, vision is intact from the day of birth. They are able to see approximately the distance between their mother's face and elbow, which is the distance that exists when feeding occurs. A newborn infant should be able to focus on her mother's (or father's) face within a few hours of birth.[51]

You may notice that your baby's eyes will occasionally roll out of focus and appear to be out of line. This is a normal occurrence in the first few months of life. At about age five to six weeks, your baby will begin to get some control over her eye muscles, and they should remain perfectly aligned by six months.[40] If you ever notice a stray or "lazy eye" in your baby after this age, this needs to be evaluated immediately!

Subconjunctival Hemorrhages

These are red marks on the whites of the eyes that occur during the pushing stage of labor when some pressure is placed on the baby's head. The marks represent small amounts of blood under the thin covering, or conjunctiva, of the eye and do not affect vision.

Common Occurrences During The First Year

Narrow Tear Ducts

Some parents of newborns are concerned that one, or both, of their baby's eyes is always watery. After being evaluated by a medical provider and being assured that there is no infection, your child may be diagnosed with narrow tear ducts.

The tear ducts are located on the lower inner eyelid and are responsible for the drainage of tears from the eyes. In some babies, this duct is small or occasionally becomes blocked and the tears back up.

Most eye specialists will wait until a baby is one year of age before performing a simple procedure to open this duct up some, as it usually does so on its own as the child grows. Ask your medical provider to show you how to massage the tear duct to keep it flowing freely and prevent blockage and back up.

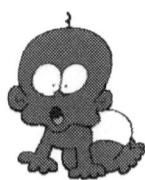

> Please let your medical provider know if the whites of your baby's eyes become red or yellow or the pupil (black center of eye) appears cloudy.

Conjunctivitis (Pink-Eye)

Pink-eye is the common name for conjunctivitis. It is so-called because the affected eye usually becomes pink (and sometimes even red) in color.

A child with pink-eye will typically wake up in the morning or after a long nap with her eye crusted shut, as the eye discharge has not been able to flow freely while she was laying down. This is a highly contagious infection and usually will be seen in both eyes if the child rubs one eye and then the other with the same hand.

In infants the infection may be due to chlamydia. If this is the case then an antibiotic eye ointment will be prescribed. In older infants, the infection can be due to a virus or bacteria and it is not always easy to tell the difference. Your medical provider will be able to examine your child to determine if antibiotic eye drops are needed.

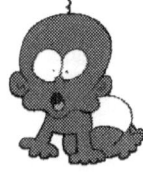

> Please call your medical provider if you notice that the skin surrounding the eyes becomes red or swollen, or if the eye seems to be "popping out" from the socket.

Common Occurrences During The First Year

Nevus of Ota

This is just the technical name for a birthmark in the eye. These spots are blue-black in color and are not the sign of any underlying eye-disease. Nevi of Ota are more common in African-Americans than Caucasians.[51] No intervention is needed, but if you notice any change in their appearance, have your child evaluated.

Eye Color

Many infants are born with eyes that are lighter in color than they will eventually be. Eye color can continue to change until about six years of age, and, interestingly, can continue to change until adulthood in about 10% of all people.[40]

Ears

Hearing

The Joint Committee on Infant Hearing (JCIH) released a position statement in the year 2000 regarding the implementation of hearing screening in newborn infants.[19] This statement points out that before the recommendation for universal newborn testing, the average age of detection of hearing loss was 30 months (two and a half years of age).

The early detection of hearing loss allows for earlier interventions on the infant's behalf. Studies have shown that children with hearing loss or deafness are behind their "hearing" counterparts for age in many areas, including social and emotional development,. The end result may be the achievement of lower employment and educational levels as adults. JCIH recommends that all children with confirmed hearing loss or deafness begin appropriate interventions by the sixth month of life.[19]

Ear Pits and Tags

Ear pits are very common among family members. If your baby has one, look around at other relatives and you will likely note that they have one as well. An ear pit is a small passageway under the skin immediately in front of the upper ear. This passage usually ends blindly but can sometimes fill with fluid and become an infected cyst. If this happens, an ear, nose and throat

(ENT) specialist will perform a simple surgery to remove the passageway and cyst. Most people, however, experience no problems from an ear pit.

An ear tag is an actual piece of flesh that can be present in front of the ear. Ear tags range in size from barely perceptible to very large. Ear tags can be associated with hearing and kidney abnormalities, neither of which is associated with ear pits. If your baby has one, be sure that a hearing test and ultrasound of the kidneys are done before she leaves the hospital.

Otitis Media (Ear Infection)

Earache is a common complaint encountered by many medical professionals caring for pediatric patients. During the first year of life, most children will experience one or two ear infections.

The pain of an ear infection is due to the buildup of pus and pressure behind the eardrum. Occasionally, the eardrum will "pop" and the pus will drain from the ear canal. Although this seems frightening, the child usually feels better afterwards, as the pressure and pain have resolved.

If the eardrum does not rupture, the child will appear crankier with any action that increases pressure in the affected ear such as sucking on a bottle or laying flat.

Ear infections can be treated with antibiotics, although some healthcare providers use a "watchful waiting" approach. Some ear infections are actually caused by viruses and do not respond to antibiotics. Viral ear infections will clear on their own over a period of several days.

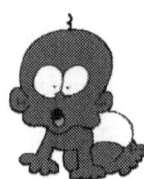

> Please call your child's medical provider if you notice that the back of the ear is red and swollen, or that the ear is pushed out and away from face. These are signs that the ear infection has spread to the bone behind the ear.

Common Occurrences During The First Year

Nose

Milia

Milia appear as little yellow bumps on the nose of a newborn infant. Milia are due to the effects of a mother's hormones that have passed over to the baby through the umbilical cord, and resolve slowly on their own over the course of several months.

Nasal Congestion

Congestion of a baby's nose causes much anxiety for many parents. An infant is not yet able to blow her nose to clear all of the mucous and it can be quite frustrating to see a baby trying so hard to breathe through a stuffed-up nose.

For the most part, I do not recommend or prescribe decongestants for infants as the side effects can be unpredictable. Using salt-water nose drops and a bulb-suction can usually suffice to clear the baby's nose.

Try to resist the urge to repeatedly suction out the baby's nose. Constant insertion of the bulb tip into the nose can cause irritation and swelling of the baby's nasal passages, making things worse!

Mouth

Epstein's Pearls

These are white patches that can be seen in the roof of the mouth in infants. They are simply collections of fluid under the skin of that area, are not infections and do not need to be treated. The passage of time cures these quite easily.

Teething

In addition to all of the other things that your baby has to do in the first few years of life (learn to eat, walk, talk, use the potty), she has the task of erupting twenty primary teeth by the age of three years![18]

Some children actually do fine throughout the teething process and seem to experience no pain at all. There are others, however, who appear to be in absolute misery. They suck and bite on everything and prefer to be to be comforted and held.

Common Occurrences During The First Year

To ease the pain of teething, offer your child a cool washcloth to chew on or a chilled, soft teething ring. Do not freeze the teething ring, as this may actually cause injury to your baby's delicate gums. Speak with your child's healthcare provider before using any over-the-counter remedies, such as pain relievers that are applied directly to the gums, acetaminophen or ibuprofen.

Sometimes, a cyst filled with fluid or blood will appear in the gum overlying the soon-to-erupt tooth. This is called an eruption cyst and is not dangerous. It should not be popped and requires no treatment.

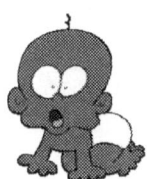

> NEVER give your baby a bone to chew on (especially chicken bones), as they may break and cause choking. In addition, although once a common folk-practice, do not rub alcohol on her gums. The alcohol will be absorbed into her system and can cause serious problems, including seizures and possible death!

Thrush

Thrush is the common name used for describing yeast infections of the mouth. These infections occur quite frequently in infants and are oftentimes seen along with yeast infections of the diaper area. The infection appears as white patches on the tongue, inner lips, gums, and inner cheeks. Thrush patches are sometimes mistaken for milk and will bleed slightly if an attempt is made to scrape them off.

Yeast infections of the mouth usually occur in younger infants due to the absence of teeth and the normal bacteria that live among them. Yeast are present naturally in an infant's mouth and may grow in an uncontrolled manner without the protective effect of these normal mouth bacteria. In older infants, the yeast may appear after antibiotics have been taken to treat another infection. These antibiotics kill off not only the infectious bacteria but the normal mouth bacteria as well, and the yeast will overgrow.

The treatment of thrush has evolved over the years. In the past, a purple dye called gentian violet was painted on the tongue to kill the yeast.

Common Occurrences During The First Year

Gentian violet stains everything that it comes into contact with purple and has basically fallen out of favor.

One commonly used medication is nystatin. This is an antifungal medication (yeast are actually fungi) that is usually squirted into each cheek four times a day for two weeks. Continue this medication for the entire duration that it has been prescribed. If discontinued too quickly, then any remaining yeast will just return.

> Boil all nipples and pacifiers at the end of each day to prevent recurrence of a thrush infection. If you are breastfeeding, rub a small amount of the medication onto your nipples before the baby feeds; this can help to keep you from getting the infection on the nipples.

Baby Bottle Tooth Decay

We have all seen cute little children who smile only to reveal rotted upper teeth. This condition, commonly known as "bottle rot," is an unfortunate occurrence as it can be prevented.

The most important preventive measure that you can take is to NEVER put your baby down to sleep with a bottle! Sleeping with a bottle allows your child's teeth to be bathed in milk, which the bacteria that normally live in the mouth will enjoy eating in addition to the underlying teeth.

Begin to brush your child's teeth from the moment they appear. This will get your baby used to the routine. There are small toothbrushes that you can buy, as well as little brushes that fit over your finger. However, just a wet cloth can be sufficient to wipe off excess food and milk.

Check to find out if the water in your community is fluorinated. If it does not contain any then your child will need fluoride supplements. The same holds true for those parents who give their children bottled water that is not supplemented with fluoride.

Toothpaste: Is It Necessary?

According to the American Dental Association, toothpaste is not necessary for children under the age of two years. Teeth can be adequately cleaned with water and friction (be it with a brush or wet cloth)[17]

Common Occurrences During The First Year

Neck and Throat

Laryngomalacia

When a baby is first born, the muscles in the larynx area of the throat are sometimes weak (referred to as "laryngomalacia"). The larynx will collapse in slightly when the baby makes an effort, such as during feeding. The result is a sound coming from the throat.

This is not suffocation and no reason for alarm. The muscles will strengthen as the baby gets older. If, however, you find that your baby appears to be choking or experiences blueness around the mouth or becomes limp, have her evaluated to be sure that there is no other problem present.

Torticollis

This term refers to a twisting of the head to one side and is commonly called "wry-neck." In a newborn infant, it can occur if the neck muscles are stretched a little during delivery. As the muscle heals, it may contract a little and pull the head to one side. You may even be able to feel a little knot where the muscle is tight.

Your baby's medical provider can show you some stretching exercises to help keep the area loose. Also, try placing visually stimulating toys or a mobile opposite the affected side, to entice the baby to look in that direction.

Chest and Lungs
Bronchiolitis

In my medical practice, almost every infant has experienced this disease at some point in her first year of life. Bronchiolitis is the general term for an infection that causes irritation and inflammation of the bronchioles in the lungs. Bronchioles are the smaller airways of the lung that lead directly to the air sacs.

Bronchiolitis is caused by several types of viruses, the most common being the respiratory syncitial virus (RSV), but also included are the influenza (flu) and rhinovirus (common-cold) viruses. These viruses incite swelling and inflammation of the lung's lower airways.

An infant's bronchiole tubes are already very small. Any inflammation decreases their size even further, leading to signs and symptoms that include a fast breathing rate, coughing and wheezing.

Bronchiolitis is often accompanied by nasal congestion, which makes breathing even more difficult. Infants are what we call "obligate nose breathers," i.e., they breathe primarily through the nose. When the nose is blocked, it is difficult for an infant to eat, as she will have to take pauses from sucking in order to catch her breath. This can cause a lowered fluid intake and lead to dehydration.

The severity of bronchiolitis can vary greatly among infants; some may only develop mild cough and a stuffy nose, whereas others develop severe trouble breathing and feeding and require hospitalization. Risk factors for the development of severe bronchiolitis include: being a young infant (less than two months of age), prematurity and underlying heart or lung disease.

Treatment of bronchiolitis is limited, as it is a viral infection so antibiotics do nothing to cure the infection or speed recovery. All interventions are made to help support the infant throughout the duration of the illness and prevent any secondary problems. For some infants, this may just be regular suctioning of the nose to help make breathing easier. For others with more severe disease, this may mean hospitalization to allow for fluids to be given through an IV and the provision of supplemental oxygen.[40]

Some infants experience an improvement of their symptoms when given albuterol, the medication used to treat asthma. This medication can help to open up the breathing tubes in the lungs. Ask your healthcare provider if it is worth trying for your baby.

Prevention is the best possible method to avoid this disease. While it is impossible to eliminate all germs from your baby's environment, you can try your best to limit exposure. Insist that <u>anyone</u> who has a cold stay away from your baby!

Common Occurrences During The First Year

Respiratory Syncitial Virus (RSV)

This virus is very well known among healthcare providers who treat premature infants. It can be deadly if these babies contract it. If you have a premature infant, make sure that you do all you can to protect her. Do not let ANYONE who is sick, even if only mildly, near her.

During RSV season, which is typically October through March, premature infants should receive a vaccination called Synagis®. The vaccine it is actually an injection of antibodies to help fight RSV infection. It must be given monthly throughout the entire RSV season. Your baby may still get the infection, but the severity of it can be greatly decreased.

The guidelines for administration of Synagis® are available from your neonatal healthcare practitioner. Enquire about this immunization before your baby leaves the neonatal intensive care unit,

Accessory Nipple

An accessory nipple is basically an extra nipple that can appear anywhere along an imaginary milk line that runs from the mid-collarbone to the foot. The extra nipple can vary in appearance, from being just a flat dark spot to a fully formed nipple and areola. Accessory nipples are eleven times more common in African-American infants than in Caucasians.[40] No intervention is needed unless there are cosmetic reasons for removal.

Breast Buds

At birth, many babies will have small amounts of breast tissue present. These breast bud are secondary to the presence of the mother's hormones in the baby's blood. The buds will slowly resolve over a period of several months. Of note, breast buds can appear in either a girl or boy infant!

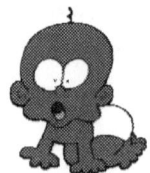

If your baby develops any redness or increased swelling over the breast area, these could be signs of a blocked milk duct that has become infected.

Abdomen and Digestive System
Vomiting

Almost all babies experience some amount of spitting-up over the first year of life. Especially during the first few months, your baby may spit-up some of her milk when she is burped or sits too upright immediately after eating. Anything that increases pressure in the stomach will cause some milk to come back up, because the muscles that control the entry of food in the stomach are still relatively weak. With time, this will resolve, and the only concern you will really have is making sure to always carry a change of clothes for the baby!

Vomiting, on the other hand, is different from spitting-up. The cause of vomiting varies based on the age of the child. If your child appears to be bringing up all of her milk after a feeding then that is something that needs to be addressed.

Signs of an underlying problem that is causing the vomiting include poor weight-gain, vomiting that shoots across the room, or a greenish color to the vomit. If you have any concerns that your baby is doing more than just "spitting-up", have her evaluated immediately.

Umbilical hernia

An umbilical hernia is sometimes called an outie because the belly button has a pushed-out appearance. This type of hernia is common in African-American infants and causes much concern in many parents and relatives. The condition itself is harmless, and most surgeons will wait until a child is 5 years old before fixing it.

An umbilical hernia results from the failure of the stomach muscles below the belly button to close and some of the intestines push through (this really is not as bad as it sounds). The hernia should be able to be pushed back through the hole in the muscle and it may protrude even more when the baby cries or strains.

There is no need to apply anything over the area (for example, taping a quarter, or wrapping the baby's waist with cloth or gauze). In fact, some children have developed infections under coins that have been taped to their

Common Occurrences During The First Year

abdomens with the hope of pressing the hernia into place.

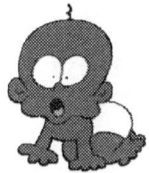

> Have your child examined immediately if the hernia appears stuck, swollen, red, or painful.

Diarrhea

The definition of diarrhea is very general, as bowel movement patterns vary greatly among people. "Normal" is what is considered normal for the child in question.

Breast-fed babies usually have loose, seedy, mustard-colored bowel movements each time that they are fed. Formula-fed babies may have a bowel movement once or twice a day. Once your baby develops her bowel-movement pattern, you will know what is normal for her. As long as the movements are not painful and do not contain blood, then your child is probably okay.

Diarrhea is defined as an increase in the frequency and a decrease in the consistency of the child's normal bowel movements. Diarrhea has many causes, and the treatment will depend on the underlying cause.

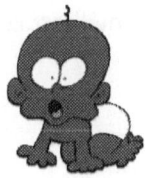 Call your child's healthcare provider immediately if your child has chalky, clay-colored or bloody bowel movements.

Constipation

On the flip side of diarrhea is constipation. The definition of constipation can cause as much confusion as that of diarrhea. Again, what is important is your child's individual pattern of bowel movements.

Some babies (in fact, most) will have a bowel movement immediately after each feeding due to a reflex called the "gastro-colic reflex." This reflex is very strong in infants and triggers the bowel movement as soon as milk enters the baby's stomach.

There are some babies, however, who may go less often. Some breast-fed infants may go several days without having a bowel movement. It is thought that in these infants, the milk is so well absorbed that there really is no waste left to eliminate

As long as the bowel movements are soft when your baby does go, there probably is no concern. However, if there is a sudden change in your baby's bowel movement patterns, or you are concerned, do not hesitate to have her examined.

One common concern that I encounter in the office with parents of newborn infants is that the baby seems to be in pain and straining to move her bowels. When the baby does finally have a bowel movement, it is very soft, and yellowish in color. This is not constipation. What looks to be pain and straining is actually just the baby using all of her strength to push.

Some babies do develop constipation and if it is present, a search must be made for the cause. In the past, people have blamed the iron in formula with constipating their child and switched to low iron formula. Under no circumstances should you do this. It can result in severe anemia in the baby. There are other dietary changes that can be made which can be very effective. These include adding prunes or prune juice. Occasionally, the use of a glycerin suppository may be necessary. Do not do any of these interventions without first finding out why your baby is constipated.

Reflux

Most infants will have some degree of reflux early on, which just refers to the flow of milk back up from the stomach and to the esophagus (the tube leading from the mouth to the stomach). As mentioned above in the section on vomiting, there is a muscle controlling entry into the stomach that is not completely functional at birth. Over time, the muscle strengthens, and the episodes of reflux should decrease.

Some infants are referred to as "happy spitters." They vomit after feeding, but their growth is not affected. They are keeping enough milk down to have the calories needed to grow. In others, the vomiting is so severe that the baby does not gain weight as expected and it is in these cases that medical interventions are made.

Any baby diagnosed with reflux should have a study called an "upper-GI" to be sure that there are no other problems that are causing the vomiting. In this study, the baby drinks a dye (it is safe) and an X-ray is taken of her stomach. This will outline the shape of the stomach, esophagus and, sometimes, the small intestine.

If your baby has reflux that is severe enough to affect her growth, then treatment is needed. Medical treatment includes medications to lower the acid content of the stomach to prevent damage to the esophagus when the baby has reflux episodes. There are also modifications that can be made regarding feeding. Some healthcare providers recommend thickening the baby's feeds with rice cereal. You can also try maintaining the baby in a semi-upright position for approximately 45 minutes after feeding. Laying flat facilitates the flow of milk back up into the esophagus and being too upright puts pressure on the stomach and works to help push the milk back up as well.

Some infants have silent reflux, a condition in which the baby has episodes of reflux that do not reach the mouth and therefore vomiting is not seen. These babies may show other signs and symptoms including constant cough and wheeze (from milk entering the lungs), a hoarse cry (from irritation of the vocal cords by the acid-containing milk that is refluxed) and just general crankiness.

In cases of uncertainty regarding the diagnosis of reflux, there are tests that can be done in the hospital setting in which a probe is inserted through the nose and into the stomach. The probe is kept in place for approximately twenty-four hours during which it will be able to detect and keep a record of any reflux episodes.

Extremities (Arms and Legs)
Positional molding

Positional molding refers to a temporary change in the appearance of the baby due to space constraints in the womb during pregnancy. Depending on how the baby is laying in the womb, different parts of her body can be pressed into a position that remains for some time after birth. These changes are temporary, and over the first few months of life outside of the womb, the "molded" part will return to its normal shape.

The most commonly seen molding of a baby's lower body are "pigeon-toes" and "bow-legs." The mainstay of treatment is basically watching the baby over time to be sure that the affected body part returns to its normal position.

Common Occurrences During The First Year

Extra digits

Some children are born with "supernumerary digits," or extra fingers or toes. These extra appendages can range from a small stub attached by a band of skin to a fully formed finger or toe attached by bone. Depending on the extent of the attachment, surgery may be needed for removal. Most healthcare practitioners recommend that a plastic surgeon perform the removal, in order that the best cosmetic result is obtained.

Skin

Skin Color

In my family, I jokingly comment that each baby is like a roll of the dice. We range in hue from French vanilla to decadent mocha with all shades in-between.

Most persons who identify themselves as African-American come from a very deep gene pool, reflective of the varied mixings through the years between our African ancestors and almost every other ethnicity!

Interestingly, there are actually four proteins in the skin that are responsible for pigmentation, or skin color. Nearly everyone has heard of melanin, the pigment that gives skin a brown-black color. Did you know, though, that there are also yellow, red and blue pigments that make up our coloring? In a darker-hued person, these other pigments may be harder to see, but they are there.

Melanin is produced by special cells that are located in the upper layers of the skin called melanocytes. After production, melanin is shipped out in a tiny package called a melanosome. In the melanosome, melanin is colorless, but it is packaged along with a protein that processes it to varying degrees of intensity. The degree to which this processing occurs determines how lightly or darkly pigmented a person will be.[63]

In a newborn baby, the skin color is usually not completely developed. Most people will look back at their newborn infant's first photo and wonder who it is. Over the process of several months, your baby will reach her genetically determined skin tone.

A commonly known fact is that melanin provides protection of the skin from the ultraviolet (UV) radiation that is present in sunlight. There is a misconception, however, that darker-skinned persons are safe from UV exposure due to higher amounts of melanin in their skin and that they do not need sunscreen. This is absolutely not true and, in fact, dangerous to believe. No matter what a person's skin color is, she must use sun block to prevent damage to the skin cells and possible skin cancer.

> When taking your baby out in the sun, dress her in clothes that will shield her skin from UV rays. Sunscreen is not recommended for infants under six months of age, so it is best to keep them out of the sun altogether. Once over this age, begin to use a sunscreen with an SPF (Sun Protection Factor) of at least 15. Apply the sunscreen 30 minutes before outdoor play, and every 2 to 3 hours thereafter.[36]

Newborn Rashes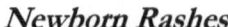

The skin of a newborn infant is rarely the perfection seen in advertisements. Following is a list of the more common, normal rashes that can be seen in newborn infants. These rashes do not require treatment and will resolve on their own with time. However, if you notice any rash that concerns you, please have your child evaluated by her medical provider to be sure that it is a normal rash and not a sign of infection

ʚɞ **Congenital Pustular Melanosis**

- Seen more commonly in children of color, this rash exists in three distinct phases. Some children are born with the rash present, and others may develop it in the days following birth.[63]
- Phase one consists of a pimple-like bump called a pustule, which can appear to be filled with pus. Rest-assured, this is not an infection and no treatment is needed.
- The second phase occurs when the pustule resolves and a scaly ring remains, with a freckle in the middle.

Common Occurrences During The First Year

- The third, and final, phase is the freckle, which will fade over time.

ଔ Erythema Toxicum Neonatorum

- This rash is not present at birth, but rather develops over the first few days of life outside of the womb. It generally appears as red splotches with a white center.[63] Of note, the rash can come and go, and can appear more intense in areas of warmth, such as the legs after having been covered by clothing.

ଔ Neonatal (Baby) Acne

- This form of acne is thought to be secondary to the hormones that were passed from the mother to the baby through the umbilical cord. Over the course of about three months, these hormones are metabolized and removed from the baby's circulation.

- Never use over-the-counter acne products on an infant. A baby's skin is much thinner than that of an adult, so these

211

medications will have a harmful effect on your infant's skin.

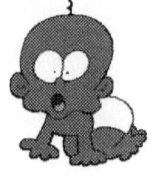

> Let your medical care provider know **immediately** if your baby develops any bumps filled with clear fluid; this could be a sign of herpes infection, whether or not you are known to have it.

Birth marks

☙ Café-au-lait spots

Very common in African-American infants, these birthmarks get their name for their appearance of being "café-au-lait", or "coffee-with-milk" colored. The incidence in African-American infants is approximately 120/1000, compared with that of 3/1000 in Caucasian infants.[51]

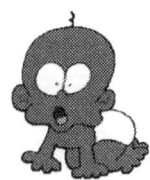

> If you notice that your baby has a large number of these birthmarks, let your healthcare provider know. It could be a sign of an underlying nervous-system disorder.

Common Occurrences During The First Year

ଔ Mongolian Spots

- Seen most commonly in children of color (African-American, Asian, Latino), these bluish patches of skin color usually appear over the lower back. They can be quite large, and can also be located in other places over the back or other parts of the body.

- Over time, these marks tend to fade, and the baby's skin color blends in more, making them appear less noticeable.

Diaper Rashes
ଔ Irritant

- The environment created in a diaper is one that can facilitate the development of an irritant rash. Even if you change your baby's diaper every hour, some infants have more sensitive skin than others, and a rash may still occur.

- Consider applying an emollient barrier to protect the skin (products containing petrolatum or zinc oxide). Letting the diaper area dry naturally in the air helps, but can be a bit risky, as your baby has no control of when she will pee or poop!

ೞ Yeast

- In some cases of diaper rash, the skin becomes extremely red and inflamed and you may notice red bumps around the border. If this is the case, your baby may have a yeast infection.

- This infection is **NOT** the same as the vaginal yeast infections seen in women and can develop in both little boys and girls in diapers. The warm, moist and dark environment created in the diaper area provides optimum growth conditions for candida, a yeast that normally lives on the skin.

- Treatment will require application of a preparation containing anti-fungal ingredients, which can be obtained by prescription.

Common Occurrences During The First Year

Eczema

Also called "atopic dermatitis", eczema is a skin condition in which dry patches develop in areas throughout the body. In infants, these patches are usually more apparent on the face (cheeks) and creases of the arms and legs.

Occasionally, you will need to use an unscented, non-allergenic soap and perfume free lotions, in case of sensitivity to conventional baby products. You may also notice that the eczema flares after eating certain foods. Your doctor may suggest an elimination diet, in which the food in question is eliminated to see if the skin improves.

> In order to avoid possible nutritional deficiencies, do not try an elimination diet to treat eczema without the supervision of your child's healthcare provider.

For many years, steroid creams and ointments have been used to control the dry, red patches of eczema. These creams should not be used for extended periods of time as they can cause a weakening of the skin to which they have been applied. They also should not be applied to large surface areas of an infant's body, as they can become absorbed into the blood stream and cause side effects. There are also non-steroid-based creams available. Your baby's medical care provider can work with you to decide which products are best for your child.

There are some interventions that you can make to help prevent eczema flares and keep your baby more comfortable. Apply a moisturizer (preferably fragrance free, non-allergenic) to your infant's skin right after bathing her and before toweling her completely off. This will allow for a moist layer between the skin and the moisturizer and will slow down the drying-out process.

You can also elect to bathe your baby every-other-day. Some parents have found this suggestion to be downright nasty, as they would consider it to be very uncleanly to not bathe every day. When your child is younger, though, she will not be getting very dirty. For the health of her skin, it may be better to skip a day. Bathing can dry out the skin, which can be made even worse with the rubbing motion of towel-drying.

Finally, make sure that you wash your baby's clothing in a mild detergent made specifically for infants or one that is perfume and dye-free.

Cradle Cap

Cradle cap is another condition thought to be associated with the presence of the mother's hormones in the baby's system for the first few months of life.

Cradle cap can range in appearance from a few flakes on the scalp to a full blown case of thick, yellow, crusty scales adhering to the scalp with a reactionary red, greasy rash on the face, behind the ears and the diaper area. The condition can even progress to cracking and bleeding of the affected area, which is very uncomfortable for the baby.

Contrary to popular belief, the flakes on the scalp are due to overproduction of oil and not dryness. It used to be recommended that the scalp be oiled, but this can actually make things worse by plugging up the pores of the scalp.

Most healthcare providers will prescribe a sulfur-containing shampoo, which works well to decrease the flaking, along with a mild steroid-based cream or ointment to apply to the affected skin areas. Like other hormone-associated changes in your baby, the condition should improve as her body eliminates your hormones from her system.

> In severe cases of cradle cap, the application of baby oil to soften the scales with subsequent removal of the scales using a soft brush or toothbrush will improve the appearance.

Common Occurrences During The First Year

Heart and Circulatory System

The human body has an intricate system of cells living in a fluid environment. Taken together, these components of the body form blood. There are some disorders of the blood cells that are seen more commonly in persons of African descent, such as sickle-cell anemia and G6PD deficiency. There are also disorders that primarily affect the blood that are common in children in general, including anemia and lead poisoning.

Heart Murmurs

Telling parents that their child has a heart murmur often causes unnecessary fear, although this response is understandable. Most people have heard a story of someone who had a heart murmur and ended up with some serious heart condition.

The first thing to understand is that a heart murmur is just a sound that the medical provider hears when listening to the heart. In children, many murmurs are "innocent," and are due to the medical provider's being able to hear the flow of blood through a normal heart. Children have very little fat and muscle on their chest walls so it is easier to hear this normal blood flow than in an adult.

On occasion, the heart murmur may be due to blood flow through an abnormality in the heart. Even if an abnormality is present, it may be a mild one and no intervention will be needed. Most medical providers will refer a child with a heart murmur that sounds outside the range of normal limits to a pediatric cardiologist (heart specialist) for evaluation and reassurance.

> Children who have severe heart defects usually show other problems, such as difficulty breathing, eating and growing due to the physical demands on the heart.

Blood
❀ Sickle Cell Anemia
What is it?

The red blood cells in our bodies are responsible for carrying oxygen to our organs and tissues. There is a protein called hemoglobin that is normally present in groups of four in each red blood cell. Hemoglobin has a carrying site for loading and unloading oxygen.

In sickle cell anemia, there is a mutation that causes an abnormal hemoglobin molecule to be formed. This hemoglobin is less effective at carrying oxygen. In addition, it causes the red blood cell to change from a normal, donut shape to a "sickle" shape, hence the term sickle cell anemia.

These abnormally shaped red blood cells can become stuck in the small blood vessels of the body, causing problems such as stroke, bone pain and pneumonia.

Types of sickle-cell

There are many different mutations that can occur to the gene code for hemoglobin, resulting in many different hemoglobin variants. A person needs to have two copies of this abnormal genetic code in order to have the actual sickle cell disease.

People who have only one copy of the abnormal hemoglobin gene are considered to have sickle cell trait, and can pass it on to their own children. When two people with sickle cell trait have a child, there is a 25% chance that the child will be born with sickle cell anemia, 25% chance that she will have completely normal hemoglobin, and 50% chance that she will have the trait.

Why?

It is thought that sickle cell trait actually allows people with the blood disease malaria to do better than people with normal hemoglobin.[30]

The parasite that causes malaria attacks red blood cells because it needs oxygen to grow. The oxygen content in a sickle cell is lower than that in normal red blood cells. Historically, this meant that in areas where the incidence of malaria is high (such as in Africa), individuals with the sickle cell trait actually had a better chance of survival than those without it, thereby passing their genetic codes on to the next generation.

Treatment

There is no treatment necessary for sickle-cell trait. It is important to be aware, however, that the measures of hemoglobin done when testing for iron-deficiency anemia will run lower than average. Individuals with sickle-cell trait may be erroneously diagnosed with iron-deficiency anemia and prescribed iron replacement therapy when it is really not needed. This can be dangerous over the long-term, as iron can build up in the liver and lungs and cause long-term secondary problems.

Children who have sickle cell anemia require intensive medical attention at regular intervals to anticipate and prevent problems. This medical care should ideally be provided by a team lead by a pediatric hematologist (blood specialist).

✺ G6PD Deficiency

This is a condition of the red blood cell as well. There is an enzyme, glucose-6-phosphate dehydrogenase (G6PD), that functions to protect the red blood cells from chemical stress that occurs after certain substances are consumed. These substances include medications (aspirin, sulfa drugs, anti-malarial drugs), foods (fava beans) and chemicals (naphthalene, found in moth balls). When the above substances gain access to the blood stream, the red blood cells that are G6PD deficient are destroyed and a rapid, serious anemia will occur.

There are two main types of G6PD deficiency: one found primarily in persons of Mediterranean descent and the other, in persons of African descent. It is important that at-risk children be tested for this blood cell disorder. Severe anemia can be prevented simply by avoiding the medications and substances that can cause problems in a G6PD-deficient individual.

In some states, expanded newborn screens are done, and the test for this deficiency may be included. If not, ask your healthcare provider to have your child tested. It is a simple blood test, and can be done at the time of other routine blood tests (lead, anemia).

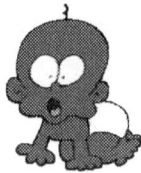

> If your child has G6PD deficiency, let her healthcare provider know immediately if you notice that she has yellowing of the skin or eyes.

Common Occurrences During The First Year

☙ Anemia

Anemia is not a disease in and of itself. It is a symptom of another problem that has the end result of lowering the amount of hemoglobin available for carrying oxygen throughout the body.

Most of the symptoms of anemia are due to decreased oxygen delivery to the body. These include fatigue, pale skin and, in young children, behavioral problems.

The most common cause of anemia in young children is iron-deficiency anemia. Children are at risk for this type of anemia for several reasons:

- Iron received from Mom during pregnancy runs out by about 6 months of age
- They tend to be picky eaters
- Cow's milk is low in iron content

How does low iron cause anemia?

Iron is needed by the body to make hemoglobin. Hemoglobin is charged with carrying and delivering oxygen throughout the body. When iron stores are low, there is decreased production of hemoglobin and, therefore, decreased oxygen levels in the body.

Diagnosis

Finding out if your child has anemia is very simple. There are finger-stick hemoglobin tests that can be done to determine the level immediately, or blood can be taken directly from your child's vein and sent out for analysis. This test is usually done between 9 and 12 months of age at the routine child health exam.

Treatment

There are several steps to the successful treatment of iron deficiency anemia. First, the body's iron stores must be replaced. This is done with prescription iron preparations. Brush your child's teeth after giving the vitamins, to prevent staining.

You can also make some dietary changes to increase the iron content of the foods that your child eats. These dietary changes should continue well past the completion of iron replacement therapy, in order to prevent the recurrence of anemia. The following is a list of iron-rich foods to incorporate into your child's diet.[38]

Common Occurrences During The First Year

> **Iron-Rich Foods**
> Red meat
> Dark poultry
> Salmon
> Eggs
> Tofu
> Enriched grains
> Dried beans/peas
> Dried fruits (raisins)
> Leafy green vegetables
> Iron-fortified cereals
>
> If your child is vegetarian, pay special attention to providing high iron and iron-fortified foods.

Prevention

Do not feed your baby whole cow's milk before the end of the first year, as the iron content is too low. Some children are also unable to digest whole cow's milk in the first year of life. This can lead to damage of the walls of the intestine with slow, chronic blood loss. Over time, this blood loss will lead to anemia.

There is some controversy over whether breastfed infants need iron supplementation. The levels of iron in breast milk are lower than those in cow's milk; however, the iron in breast milk is much more easily absorbed. Discuss with your healthcare provider whether or not iron supplements are needed.

○8 Lead Poisoning

Lead has a long history of use that can be traced all of the way back to Egyptian times. Of most concern to our children's health is the history of use of lead-based paints and leaded gasoline in our country. This has left a large storehouse of lead in the environment.[4.26]

Many people believe that if they live in a brand new home then their children are safe and protected from lead exposure. The fact is lead is present in more places than people realize. Lead dust has accumulated in soil over the years and the concentration can be quite high in some locations.

The concerns about lead poisoning are with good reason. Lead has been shown to cause problems in the developing brain as well as behavioral disturbances, stomach upset and even nervous system disease. It is for all of these reasons that screening should be done for all children at a young age. Most medical providers check blood lead levels at age 9 to 12 months and then based on risk thereafter.

> Be sure that your child's lead level is obtained from venous blood (taken directly from a vein) and not a finger-stick sample. Finger-stick lead levels are often falsely elevated due to the presence of lead dust on the finger.

If your child is diagnosed with an elevated lead level, it is important that every area in which she spends time be evaluated as a possible source. This includes grandparents' homes and daycare settings. The following page lists some common sources of lead.

> **Sources of Lead**[4,26]
>
> Drinking water (from lead pipes)
>
> Imported toys, jewelry, and candy (especially from Mexico)
>
> Work involving automobile batteries
>
> Some home-health remedies
>
> Pottery
>
> Lead-based paint
>
> Some cosmetics (kohl)

Prevention of lead exposure is key. The medications needed to lower blood lead levels are not without their side effects. One of the most important things that you can do to prevent lead poisoning is to optimize your child's diet.

Make sure that your child eats foods that are rich in calcium. Calcium competes with lead in the stomach for absorption. Iron also inhibits lead absorption from the stomach so include foods rich in this nutrient as well. Know, however, that calcium and iron compete with each other's absorption into the blood. Try to give these foods at separate meal times.

Common Occurrences During The First Year

Genital Systems

Male

When a medical provider performs the very first exam on a newborn boy, she checks to make sure that all of the parts are there and functioning.

Some newborn boys have fluid in the scrotum right after birth, giving it a full look. Both testicles should be in the scrotum although, at times, they can be "retractile." Retractile testes are both present but move up and down from the scrotum and into the groin. Finally, the urethra (the opening from which urine exits) should be in the very center of the glans (head of the penis).

There has been recent discussion regarding the need to routinely circumcise newborn boys. In some cultures circumcision is a religious rite; in others, it is done to allow the child to look like other males in the family who have been circumcised. The American Academy of Pediatrics (AAP) has issued a policy statement in which they did a comprehensive review of the medical literature regarding the circumcision of newborn males.[2] They concluded that there may be some benefits to circumcision of newborn males including decreased risk of urinary tract infections and, later, the contraction of HIV.

The current published medical evidence does not support a universal recommendation to circumcise. Instead, the AAP suggests that parents be given a choice using all of the current information available to aide in this decision-making process. Finally, they suggest that if a circumcision is done, adequate pain relief be provided to the infant as there are safe, effective medications available for that purpose.

Female

Most of a girl's reproductive organs are located internally. However, the medical provider can and should examine the external appearance. Some girls are born with an imperforate hymen. This means that the hymen has no opening to allow for the passage of menstrual blood and other vaginal secretions.

Common Occurrences During The First Year

You may notice that your infant girl has a white vaginal discharge in the first week or so after she is born. There may even be mild bleeding, sometimes called a "pseudo-period". These are all both secondary to her body withdrawing from the hormones that you passed to her across the placenta.

Urinary Tract Infection

Children with urinary tract infections do not show the classic symptoms that are seen in adults (frequent, painful urination). They will usually only show high fever and, occasionally, vomiting and diarrhea. For a child who is not yet able to speak, one has to keep the possibility of such an infection in mind when there is a high fever and no source of infection is found.

There are some abnormalities that children are born with that give them a higher risk of developing urinary tract infections. A urinary tract infection in an infant automatically requires a search for developmental problems of the urinary tract. The evaluation should be performed by a physician who specializes in child urology. The underlying goal is to prevent recurrent urine infections.

> Multiple infections of the urine can cause kidney scarring and early high blood pressure due to kidney damage.

Hernia

The type of hernia discussed here is different from the umbilical hernia discussed earlier. This type of hernia is called an inguinal hernia and can be seen in boys and girls, although they are more common in boys.

During normal development, the testicles of a boy are located in the abdomen. As the baby reaches the time for his delivery, the testicles will come down out of the abdomen and pass into the scrotum through a passageway called the inguinal canal. Sometimes, the opening to this canal does not close completely, allowing for part of the intestine to travel through.

Most hernias can slide up and down through the hole in the canal. On occasion, the hernia can become stuck in the canal. This results in its blood supply being cut off and is an emergency situation. If you notice any bulge in the testicle or along the groin area, seek immediate attention. It is best to fix the problem before it becomes an emergency.

Girls can also get hernias, and theirs appear through a defect in the lower groin area. These defects should be fixed in the same way that they would be in a little boy.

General Health Concerns

Crying

Who hasn't heard of that lucky parent who has a good baby? This baby only cries when hungry or in need of a diaper change. She slept through the night from day one. When she is awake, she is just a happy little tyke full of smiles and coos for her parents. This ideal child has become the hope of many prospective parents who dread the thought of spending long nights awake with their infant.

I would like to begin this section by affirming that there is no such thing as a "good baby." Infants are born with their personalities already intact. When your child comes into the world, you will be involved in a constant learning process of how she responds to her internal needs and stimuli.

Some infants truly do not cry much and, in fact, may need to be awakened every few hours because, left to their own devices, they would sleep for hours on end and miss some of their feedings. Then, there is the other end of the spectrum. The infant who cries and cries and does not calm with

Common Occurrences During The First Year

the usual interventions: changing, feeding, rocking and soothing. These are the children that can be challenging, especially for parents who are not prepared.

Infant crying patterns vary from one child to the next. One study found that two month-old infants cry an average of 105 minutes in a twenty-four hour period. This amount increases to 165 minutes per day by six weeks of age, and then decreases to less than sixty minutes per day by twelve weeks of age.[54]

> In 3-week-old infants, crying is more common between the time periods of 6 p.m. to 11 p.m. By six weeks of age, infants tend to cry more often from 3 p.m. to midnight.[54]

Crying is your infant's sole means of communication. It is up to you, the caregiver, to determine the cause of her distress. This can be a challenge at times. As a pediatrician, I am often presented with infants who have been crying and cranky. My approach to finding out why is to be systematic and always begin by reviewing the "usual suspects" of infant crying. This same approach can work for you as well.

Begin with the most common causes of infant crying, and work your way down. Is she:

- Sitting in a wet or soiled diaper?
- Hungry?
- Tired?
- Over stimulated?

If, after checking everything out and your baby is well with no signs of illness, it may just be that she has colic.

Common Occurrences During The First Year

Colic

Many healthcare providers use the "rule of 3's" as a guideline to differentiation between normal and excessive infant crying:

- ~ Occurring by the 3 rd week of life
- ~ Lasting for at least 3 hours a day
- ~ Occurring more than 3 days in one week
- ~ Resolves by 3 months of age

I know all too well the feelings of frustration that a parent with a colicky baby can feel. When he was three weeks old, my first son cried, religiously, from ten pm until three am. Convinced SOMETHING had to be wrong, I took a trip to the emergency room only to arrive and present the doctor with a calm, peacefully sleeping infant. After a thorough examination, I was told that my baby had colic and not to worry, that this would all pass by the time he was 12 weeks old.

This child is now 10 years old, and his nights of crying have long passed

(See Appendix A for information on the book :The Happiest Baby on the Block" for excellent tips o calming a colicky baby).

Shaken Baby Syndrome[3,24]

Shaken baby syndrome is the unfortunate outcome of the shaking of a child when a parent or caregiver loses control. The damage is done when a child is taken by the shoulders and shaken back and forth, allowing the head to roll around on the neck. The delicate blood vessels in the infant's brain tear, followed by serious bleeding into the brain and skull.

If at ANY point you feel that you may hurt your child, please, ask for help. Shaken baby syndrome causes severe brain damage from which recovery is rare, and can even cause death. If your child is crying and there is nothing you can do to make her stop, put her in a safe place (crib or bassinette) and take a ten-minute break.

Common Occurrences During The First Year

Sudden Infant Death Syndrome

Sudden infant death syndrome, or SIDS, is defined as "a sudden death in an infant in which no cause of death can be identified after a thorough investigation."[40] This death usually occurs between the ages of one and five months, is more frequent in male infants, and has a **two to three times increased incidence in African-American infants** as compared with whites.[16]

There are factors that have been associated with an increased risk of SIDS, some of which are modifiable by a change in behavior. These factors include: male sex of the infant, young maternal age, maternal smoking or alcohol use, and bottle-feeding.[16]

> Exposure to tobacco smoke increases a baby's risk of dying from SIDS by almost three times over baseline.

The current recommendation is to lay your baby "Back-to-Sleep," unless otherwise directed by your physician. Many parents have expressed concern that their baby may vomit and choke if she lies flat on her back; this has not been proven, but an increased risk of death due to SIDS has. SIDS deaths have decreased by 40% since the "Back-to-Sleep" campaign was instituted.[16]

At what age can you stop putting your baby on her back to sleep? My recommendation has always been that if you lay your baby on her back and she rolls onto her stomach by herself, then she is probably okay to sleep that way.

Co-sleeping

The topic of co-sleeping has been hotly debated over the past several years among experts in child healthcare and development. To date, there is no clear definition of co-sleeping. In some studies, co-sleeping refers to the practice of bed sharing, in which an infant is placed directly in the bed with an adult caretaker. In others, co-sleeping simply means that the child is within arm's reach of the adult caretaker; in this situation, the baby may be sleeping in a small crib or bassinette adjacent to the caretaker's bed.

The concern with co-sleeping in general and bed-sharing specifically is whether there may be an increased risk of sudden infant death syndrome (SIDS). James McKenna of Notre Dame University did an extensive review of the current research regarding co-sleeping and bed sharing.[46] He elaborates that before one can comment on the risks of co-sleeping, there must be a distinction between co-sleeping and bed sharing.

Dr. McKenna refers to studies that have shown that there is a difference in infant death rates between infants who bed-share with a non-smoking, non-obese, non-drug using breastfeeding mother and those who bottle-feed, smoke, are obese, use drugs, or are forced to bed-share due to poverty. Mothers in the first group tend to take precautions that include removing pillows from around the baby and placing the baby on her back to sleep (the easiest position in which to breastfeed). On the contrary, the second group tends to not exercise these precautions. He concludes that before condemning the practice of bed-sharing, one must take into consideration the context of the sharing, and that parents need to be educated on safe bed-sharing practices.

The American Academy of Pediatrics (AAP) has issued a policy statement that asserts that "bed sharing is not recommended during sleep. Infants may be brought into bed for nursing or comforting, but should be returned to their own crib or bassinette when ready to return to sleep."[16] They do note that the baby can be kept close to the mother in a separate sleeping area to facilitate breastfeeding.

If you make the decision is to bed share, only do so if you are free of drugs or alcohol, non-obese and non-smoking. Also, assure that there are no gaps between your mattress and the headboard or your mattress and the wall. Never lay your baby to sleep on top of a pillow or a soft surface (such as a waterbed) and keep all pillows and blankets away from her.

> Do not allow siblings to sleep in the same bed as your infant. Their level of awareness of the baby's presence is not as heightened as your own.
> Make sure that your partner is aware that the baby is sleeping in the bed and never leave the baby unattended on an adult bed.

Common Occurrences During The First Year

Siblings

Anyone who has a brother or sister knows that there is oftentimes competition for parental attention and affection. A small amount of this sibling rivalry is normal and healthy. Be wary, though, of an older sibling's response to the presence of a new infant in the home. Properly preparing your existing child for the new arrival can help to prevent future problems and allow for a smooth transition of the baby into the family.

The manner in which you prepare your existing child for the arrival of the new baby will depend on her current developmental stage. Toddlers and younger children have no concept of time, so telling them of the pregnancy in the earlier months may mean nothing to them. You can, of course, notify them that the baby is on the way, but you might have to remind them on a regular basis.

As your belly begins to increase in size and others can feel the baby's movements from the outside, you can include your other child even more. Let her touch your stomach, and, if possible, take her with you to a prenatal appointment. It can be very exciting to hear the heartbeat, or to see her new little brother or sister by ultrasound!

To the best of your ability, try to incorporate some special time focused only on your existing child. This will reinforce to her that although a new baby is coming, you still love her and that she is still very important to you. Let her participate in the decoration of the nursery. If possible, do not take a room away from your existing child to "give to the baby." Your child may resent and blame the baby for displacing her!

After bringing the baby home, continue to have special-time with your older child. This could be just 30 minutes of time in which she receives your complete, undivided attention.

> Consider buying a gift from the new baby to be given to her older sibling when they first meet each other in the hospital.

Common Occurrences During The First Year

For younger children, show them the appropriate way to touch the baby. Let them know that they are not to feed the baby or give her things to play with. Once your infant is more mobile and spending time playing on the floor, remind older siblings to pick up all toys after themselves. Toys made for older children usually have smaller parts that are easily inhaled and choked on by a small baby.

If you notice an extreme level or jealousy or violence towards the baby from a sibling, please do not ignore it, or expect him or her to grow out of it. There is help available, and insist that your child receive it. Waiting will only allow the resentment to become more deep-seated and difficult to resolve.

Finally, be prepared for some form of developmental regression in your older child. In some children, this just means acting more "baby-like." For others, there may be an actual loss of previous achievements, e.g. a child who was successfully potty-trained now needs diapers again. If your child responds in this manner, remember that she is not behaving this way intentionally. It is her way of returning to the time when **she** was the baby. With some patience and reassurance that she is just as important to you as the new baby is, this period will pass.

Pets and your Baby

For many families, pets were the first babies of the house. These animals become integral members of the family and can actually become jealous and territorial when you bring home your new bundle of joy!

Never underestimate the ability of your pet to become jealous and to try to harm your infant. This does not mean that you have to put it out of your home. It does mean that you should take some precautions and, if you notice that the animal is becoming overly aggressive, you may want to think about putting it up for adoption.

After your baby's birth, send one of her receiving blankets home with your support person and leave it for your pet to smell and become acquainted with. In this way, the animal can "meet" your baby before it actually sees her.

Common Occurrences During The First Year

Once you arrive home from the hospital, <u>never</u> leave the baby unattended with your pet. No matter how much you think you can trust it, your pet needs only seconds to attack and seriously injure your child. Over time, your pet will become accustomed to the new person in the house; even when that occurs, never let your guard down. Again, if the pet becomes dangerous get rid of it!

Child Care

If you decide to work outside of the home, you will need to determine who will care for your child in your absence. There has been much research into the indicators of quality childcare, and helpful guidelines are available to any parent who would like to know how to make the best possible choice.

In "A Parent's Guide to Choosing Safe and Healthy Daycare," the US Department of Health and Human Services (DHHS) outlines the following as indicators of a quality childcare program:[1]

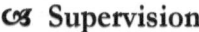

- **Supervision**
  - Are children supervised at ALL times (including during sleep)?
- **Hand washing/Diapering**
  - Is there a separate area for diapering? Are hands washed at regular intervals?
- **Director Qualifications**
- **Lead Teacher Qualifications**
- **Child: Staff Ratio and Group Size**
  - The American Academy of Pediatrics recommends a child: staff ratio of 3:1 for infants and children less than one year of age
- **Immunizations**
  - Are children in the program adequately immunized?
  - Are staff immunized and free of communicable disease?
- **Emergency plan**
  - What happens in case of emergency, such as a power outage or natural disaster?

Common Occurrences During The First Year

- **Fire Drills**
  - Are drills occurring on a monthly basis?
  - Is there a written plan?
- **Child Abuse**
  - Are all staff cleared through a child abuse background check?
- **Staff Training/First Aid**
  - Are staff trained and certified in first aid and CPR of infants and children?
- **Playground**
  - Is the play area safe and padded in case of a fall?
  - Is the area enclosed by a fence?
- **Medications**
  - Is there a medication policy for safe storage and administration?
- **Toxic Substances**
  - Are toxic substances kept out of the reach of children?

The DHHS also recommends that parents visit several different childcare providers before making a decision. Plan on staying for at least an hour to really get a feel for how the center is run.

Of particular importance for infants is the observation of safe sleeping practices. Are the caregivers following the recommendations for safe sleep, including laying babies to sleep on their backs in cribs free of blankets and stuffed toys?

> Infants who are routinely placed on their backs to sleep and then placed on their stomachs to sleep during a nap by another care provider have a 6 to 7 times increased risk of dying from SIDS![43]

Make sure that the center you choose is licensed. Licensing guidelines vary from state to state, and also among types of care providers; for example, there are different requirements for in-home versus center-based daycare. Many states also have their own certification programs, which only award certification to those childcare providers who have met certain guidelines for quality care.

Look into certification of the center by the National Association for the Education of Youth and Children (NAEYC). This organization only provides accreditation status to programs that meet their guidelines, which include: positive interactions between children and staff, continuing education for staff, respect for cultural diversity, and planned learning activities.

Baby-Proofing

I will begin this section by stating that there really is no such thing as baby-proof. Rather, we can create environments for our children that are as safe as possible by removing harmful objects to allow them to freely explore. There are, as with everything else, many products on the market to aide you in creating this safe environment, but nothing replaces supervision!

Baby-proofing begins from the minute your child is born. Make your infant's sleep area as safe as possible by always laying her on her back to sleep and keeping her crib free of blankets and stuffed toys. Even if you think that she cannot roll over, NEVER leave her unattended on a high surface such as a bed, couch or changing table. Infants have rolled off and been injured when their caregivers turned their backs thinking that the child was not yet mobile.

As your infant gets older, by about 4 months of age or so, she will begin to put everything she gets her hands on into her mouth. This means that not only do her toys have to be of a safe size but also all objects around her. Pen-caps, money, paperclips, rubber bands, really any small objects, pose a threat to your child.

At six months of age, many infants are rolling around and scooting, so the areas available for them to explore increase exponentially! Get down to your child's level, on hands and knees, and look for anything that she may be able to get her hands on.

Over the next 6 months, your child will become even more mobile. When she is able to pull to stand with support, such as on a table edge, she will be able to reach objects that were once at a distance. Keep all medications safely stored, as in an attempt to imitate you, your child may ingest them and become very ill. Cover all electrical sockets with childproof protectors, cover stove and oven controls with childproof locks and lock all cabinets to which your child may gain access. Finally, speak with all people who provide care and supervision to your child and verify that they are taking the same safety precautions as you.

> Leave out some age-appropriate toys for your child to play with. This will avoid the need to be saying "No, don't touch that," all of the time.

Fevers

Fever is one common symptom that causes great alarm in the parents of infants and young children. Fever is not a disease but an indicator that something is not right somewhere in your child's system.

Fevers are often, but not always, caused by infections. Many people will categorize fevers into low-grade and high-grade. The height of the fever **is not** a reliable indicator of the severity of the underlying illness. Some bacterial infections do not cause fevers, whereas some viral infections can cause very high fevers.

Any infant under 8 weeks of age with a fever must be evaluated by a healthcare provider. At that age, babies show very few signs of illness, so it can be difficult to tell that something is wrong; a fever may be the only clue. For older infants (older than 8 weeks of age), most healthcare providers will rely on how the child looks, as well as how well she is feeding and making diapers. A playful, active baby with a temperature of 102 degrees Fahrenheit is much less concerning than a weak, limp baby with a temperature of 100.9 degrees Fahrenheit.

When you call your provider or go into the office to be seen, be prepared to answer several questions that will help her to assess your child's condition. These questions include:

- The height of the fever
- Method by which the temperature was taken (rectal, under the arm, ear)
- Associated signs and symptoms (rashes, vomiting, diarrhea)
- Number of wet diapers
- Ill contacts (e.g. daycare, home)

Common Occurrences During The First Year

Taking Your Baby's Temperature

Either a mercury or digital thermometer can be used for taking your child's temperature. Digital thermometers will beep when the final temperature has registered. Mercury thermometers should be held in place for two minutes.

Axillary (under the arm)

Tympanic (in the ear)
Special thermometers are sold to measure the temperature in this manner. These thermometers measure the heat emitted from the eardrum.

Rectal (in the rectum)
This is the "gold-standard" of temperature taking in infants. Be careful if using a glass mercury thermometer. The end could break off in the rectum should the baby move while her temperature is being taken. Some rectal thermometers have a widened end to prevent the tip from being inserted too deeply into the rectum.

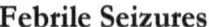

Febrile Seizures

A febrile seizure is a seizure that occurs due to the presence of a fever. These seizures occur most commonly in children aged 6 months to 5 years of age. They do not signify that the child has epilepsy.

Although these episodes are frightening for a parent or caretaker to witness, there is no actual brain damage occurring. Folk wisdom says that a spoon should be inserted into a seizing child's mouth to prevent her from swallowing her tongue. It is impossible to swallow the tongue and you may do damage by trying to do this to the child. The most important thing that you can do is to provide safe surroundings during the episode by clearing any dangerous objects from the immediate area.

Common Occurrences During The First Year

Treatment

The treatment of fever allows for a child's comfort. There are many different brand names of fever reducers available but the two main fever-reducers marketed for infants and children are acetaminophen and ibuprofen. Speak with your child's medical care provider regarding the safe dosages of these medications. Ibuprofen is not for use in infants under six months of age. Remember, the source of the fever should be determined, so be sure to have your child evaluated by her medical care provider if necessary.

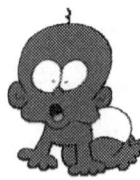

Seek immediate medical attention for any fever accompanied by a rash, difficulty eating or drinking, or excessive vomiting and diarrhea.

- Never give aspirin to a child under eighteen years of age. The use of aspirin to treat fever in children is associated with the development of a serious and sometimes fatal liver condition called Reye's Syndrome.
- Rubbing a child down with alcohol should never be done. The alcohol will be absorbed into the child's system resulting in a drop in the sugar levels, possible seizure and death.
- Do not immerse your child in a cold bath. When a person with fever is suddenly placed in cold water, the blood vessels will contract rapidly to conserve heat; this causes blood pressure to drop to dangerously low levels.

Conclusion

I do hope that you have found this book to be a worthy companion throughout your child's first year of life.

Always remember to trust your instincts when it comes to your baby's health. If you have a concern and it is not addressed then it is time to look elsewhere for a second opinion!

My ultimate goal is to create an entire series on healthcare to accompany parents and their children through each life stage, beginning from infancy and up to adulthood. Please look for these up-coming volumes, and thank you again for allowing me to be a part of your child's life.

Yours in Health,
Ena M. Cade, MD, FAAP

Appendix A

Web Resources

General Health Information

- Kid's Health   www.kidshealth.org
- Medline Plus   www.medlineplus.com
- American Academy of Pediatrics www.aap.org

Child Care Information

- National Association for the Education of Young Children www.naeyc.org

Breastfeeding

- La Leche League   www.lalecheleague.org
- African-American Breast Feeding Alliance www.aabaonline.com

Safety

- Consumer Product Safety Commission www.cpsc.gov
- National Highway Transportation Safety Administration www.nhtsa.gov

- Juvenile Products Manufacturers Administration www.jpma.org

Vaccinations

- Centers for Disease Control www.cdc.gov

Postpartum Depression

- Postpartum Support International www.postpartum.net.

Appendix B

Print Resources

The Happiest Baby on the Block: The New Way to Calm Crying and Help Your Newborn Baby Sleep Longer
Harvey Karp, MD

Blender Baby Food
Nicole Young and Nadine Day

Vaccines: What Every Parent Should Know
Paul Offit, MD and Louis Bell, MD

Nighttime Parenting (Revised): How to Get Your Baby and Child to Sleep (La Leche League International Book)
Williams Sears, MD

Vaccine Record

Vaccine	Date	Reaction	Next Due
Hepatitis B			
Hepatitis B			
Hepatitis B			
Hepatitis B			
DTaP			
DTaP			
DTaP			
DTaP			
DTaP			
Hib			
Hib			
Hib			
Hib			
IPV			
IPV			
IPV			
IPV			
Prevnar			
Prevnar			
Prevnar			
Prevnar			

Rotavirus			
Rotavirus			
Rotavirus			
MMR			
MMR			
Varivax			
Flu			
Flu			
Hepatitis A			
Hepatitis A			

References

[1] "A Parent's Guide to Choosing Safe and Healthy Childcare," Department of Health and Human Services. Accessed 10 September 2006 <http://aspe.hhs.gov>

[2] American Academy of Pediatrics. "Circumcision Policy Statement," *Pediatrics* 103(3); 686-693. March 1999

[3] American Academy of Pediatrics. Committee on Child Abuse and Neglect. "Shaken Baby Syndrome: Rotational Cranial Injuries-Technical Report." *Pediatrics* 108(1) 206-210. 1 July 2001

[4] American Academy of Pediatrics. Committee on Environmental Health. "Lead Exposure in Children: Prevention, Detection and Management." *Pediatrics* 116(4) 1036-1049. 4 October 2005

[5] American Academy of Pediatrics, Committee on Injury and Poison Prevention, "Injuries Associated With Infant Walkers" *Pediatrics* 108(3) 790-792. September 2001

[6] American Academy of Pediatrics, Committee on Public Education, "Media Education," *Pediatrics* 104(2): 341-343. August 1999

[7] American Academy of Pediatrics. Section on Breastfeeding. "Breastfeeding and the Use of Human Milk." *Pediatrics* 115(2) 496-506. 2 February 2005

[8] American Academy of Pediatrics [Syphilis] In: Pickering, LK ed. *Red Book: 2003 Report of the Committee on Infectious Diseases* 26th ed. Elk Grove, IL: AAP; 2003: 595-603

[9] American Academy of Pediatrics [Group B Streptococcus] In: Pickering, LK ed. *Red Book: 2003 Report of the Committee on Infectious Diseases* 26th ed. Elk Grove, IL: AAP; 2003: 584-593

[10] American Academy of Pediatrics [Listeriosis] In: Pickering, LK ed. *Red Book: 2003 Report of the Committee on Infectious Diseases* 26th ed. Elk Grove, IL: AAP; 2003: 405-407

[11] American Academy of Pediatrics [Varicella] In: Pickering, LK ed. *Red Book: 2003 Report of the Committee on Infectious Diseases* 26th ed. Elk Grove, IL: AAP; 2003: 595-603

[12] American Academy of Pediatrics [Hepatitis B] In: Pickering, LK ed. *Red Book: 2003 Report of the Committee on Infectious Diseases* 26th ed. Elk Grove, IL: AAP; 2003: 318-336

[13] American Academy of Pediatrics [Rubella] In: Pickering, LK ed. *Red Book: 2003 Report of the Committee on Infectious Diseases* 26th ed. Elk Grove, IL: AAP; 2003: 536-541

[14] American Academy of Pediatrics [Toxoplasma gondii infections] In: Pickering, LK ed. *Red Book: 2003 Report of the Committee on Infectious Diseases* 26th ed. Elk Grove, IL: AAP; 2003: 631-635

[15] American Academy of Pediatrics [Human Immunodeficiency Virus Infection] In: Pickering, LK ed. *Red Book: 2003 Report of the Committee on Infectious Diseases* 26th ed. Elk Grove, IL: AAP; 2003: 360-382

[16] American Academy of Pediatrics, Task Force on Infant Sleep Position and SIDS, "Changing Concepts of SIDS: Indications for Infant Sleeping Environment and Sleep Position," *Pediatrics* 105(3): 650-655. March 2000

[17] American Dental Association. ADA Statement on Early Childhood Caries. 14 March 2005. Accessed 28 July 2006 <http://www.ada.org/prof/resources/positions/statements/caries.asp>

[18] American Dental Association. Teething Copyright 1995-2006. Accessed 17 September 2006 <http://www.ada.org/public/topics/teething/asp>

[19] American Speech-Language-Hearing Association Joint Committee on Infant Hearing. Year 2000 Position Statement: Principles and Guidelines for Early Hearing Detection and Intervention Programs, c.1997-2006. Accessed 28 July 2006 <http://www.asha.org>

[20] Barclay, Laurie, Lie, Desiree, "Maternal Control of Solid Feeding Can Moderate Infant Weight Gain," *Medscape Medical News*. 11 August 2006. Accessed 18 August 2006. <http://www.medscape.com/viewarticle/542662_print>

[21] Barclay, Laurie, Lie, Desiree, "New Guidelines for Introducing Solid Foods to Avoid Development of Infant Allergies" *Medscape Medical News*. 31 July 2006. Accessed 18 August 2006.
<http://www.medscape.com/viewarticle/541952_print>

[22] Bergfeld, Wilima "Hair Care," *Dermatology Insights*, 4(1): 23-24

[23] Brooks, Jennifer, " Breastfeeding and Rickets," National Center for Policy Research for Women and Families, " 2003 June. Accessed 21 September 2006
<http://www.center4policy.org>

[24] Carbaugh, Suzanne Franklin, "Preventing Shaken Baby Syndrome." *Advanced Neonatal Care* 4(2): 118-119. 2004

[25] Centers for Disease Control and Prevention. CDC HIV/AIDS Fact Sheet, "HIV/AIDS Among Women," April 2006 <http://www.cdc.gov/hiv>

[26] Centers for Disease Control and Prevention. *National Center for Envirornmental Health Division of Emergency and Environmental Health Services*, "Childhood Lead Poisoning." 2005 May <http://www.cdc.gov/nceh/lead/lead.htm>

[27] Centers for Disease Control and Prevention, *Six Common Misconceptions about Vaccination and How to Respond to Them.* 12 May 2004. Accessed 4 August 2006 <http://www.cdc.gov/nip/publications/6mishome.htm>

[28] Centers for Disease Control and Prevention, *What Would Happen if We Stopped Vaccinations,* 19 November 2003. Accessed 24 July 2006 <http://www.cdc.gov/nip/publications/fs/gen/whatifistop.htm>

[29] Centers for Disease Control and Prevention. Fetal Alcohol Syndrome, 23 November 2005. Accessed 12 May 2006. <http://www.cdc.gov/ncbddd/fas/fasask.htm>

[30] Centers for Disease Control and Prevention. Protective Effect of Sickle Cell Trait Against Malaria-Associated Mortality and Morbidity. 23 April 2004. Accessed 31 May 2006. <http://www.cdc.gov/malaria/biology/sicklecell.htm>

[31] Centers for Disease Control and Prevention. Diabetes and Pregnancy Frequently Asked Questions. 5 October 2005. Accessed 19 May 2006. <http://www.cdc.gov>

[32] Chaudron , Linda H, "Beyond the Blues: A Guide to Understanding and Treating Prenatal and Postpartum Depression" *Birth* 31:1. 2004

[33] Consumer Product Safety Commission. A Grandparent's Guide for Family Nurturing and Safety. Accessed 2 May 2006 <http://www.cpsc.gov/cpscpub/pubs/grand/704.html>

[34] Data2010: Healthy People2010 Database, Centers for Disease Control and Prevention <http://www.cdc.gov>

[35] Davis, Katherine Finn, Parkers, Kathy P and Montgomery, Gary L, "Sleep in Infants and Young Children: Part One: Normal Sleep." *Journal of Pediatric Health* 18(2): 65-71. 2004

[36] Dowshen, Steven, Homeier, Barbara, "Sun Safety," *KidsHealth* November 2004. Accessed 28 July 2006 <http://www.kidshealth.org>

[37] "Edward Jenner," Wikipedia, 9 September 2006. Accessed 10 September 2006. <http://en.wikipedia.org/wiki/Edward_Jenner>

[38] Gavin, Mary L, "Iron and Your Child," *KidsHealth*, 2005 January. Accessed 22 May 2006. <http://kidshealth.org>

[39] Gray, John, "Hair Types," *Procter and Gamble*. Accessed 29 September 2006. <http://www.pg.com/science/haircare>

[40] Green-Hernandez, C, Singleton, Joanne K, Aronzon, Daniel Z, *Primary Care Pediatrics*, Philadelphia: Lippincott, Williams and Wilkins: 2001.

[41] Hatcher, Robert A, et al, *Contraceptive Technology*, Contraceptive Technology Communications, Inc., New York, New York: 2004

[42] "The Health Consequences of Involuntary Exposure to Tobacco Smoke: A Report of the Surgeon General, U.S. Department of Health and Human Services," <u>US Department of Health and Human Services</u>, 27 June 2006. Accessed 15 September 2006. <<u>http://www.surgeongeneral.gov/library/secondhandsmoke</u>>

[43] "Higher SIDS Risk Found in Infants Placed in Unaccustomed Sleeping Position," *NIH News*, <u>National Institutes of Health</u>, 28 February 2003. Accessed 3 October 2006

[44] Lyness, D'Arcy, Harkness, Michael, "Separation Anxiety," *KidsHealth*, July 2005. Accessed 19 September 2006. <<u>http://www.kidshealth.org</u>>

[45] March of Dimes, "Folic Acid," *Pregnancy and Newborn Health Education Center*, November 2005. Accessed 30 September 2006. <http://www.marchofdimes/com>

[46] McKenna, James J, McDade, Thomas, "Why Babies Should Never Sleep Alone: A Review of the Co-sleeping Controversy in Relation to SIDS, Bedsharing and Breast Feeding," *Pediatric Respiratory Reviews* (6):134-152. 2005

[47] "Medical Encyclopedia: Sickle Cell Anemia," Medline Plus, 13 April 2005. Accessed 19 September 2006 <http://www.nlm.nih.gov>

[48] National Heart Lung and Blood Institute. Diseases and Conditions Index, "Sarcoidosis" August 2005. Accessed 19 May 2006 <http://www.nhlbi.nih.gov/health/dci/Diseases/sarc/sar_whatis.html>

[49] National Highway Traffic Safety Administration. <u>Child Restraint Re-Use After Minor Crashes</u>. Accessed 31 May 2006 <<u>http://www.nhtsa.dot.gov</u>>

[50] National Institute of Arthritis and Musculoskeletal and Skin Diseases. <u>Lupus: A Patient Care Guide for Nurses and Other Health Professionals</u>. 2001 May. Accessed 19 May 2006. <<u>http://www.niams.nih.gov</u>>

[51] Oski, Frank A, *Principles and Practice* of Pediatrics. Philadelphia: J.B. Lippincott Company, 1990

[52] Perry, Bryce D., "Childhood Experience and the Expression of Genetic Potential: What Childhood Neglect Tells Us About Nature and Nurture," *Brain and Mind* (3):79-100, 2002

[53] Physicians Drug Reference, "Pregnancy Drug Categories," Thompson PDR, Montvale, NJ c. 2006

[54] Pray, Steven W, "Infant Colic: The Therapeutic Puzzle," *US Pharmacist* 22(3) 1997. Accessed 4 May 2006 <http://www.medscape.com/viewarticle/407594>

[55] "Pregnancy: When You Have a Chronic Health Condition," *MayoClinic.com* 1 August 2005. Accessed 19 May 2006. <http://www.mayoclinic.com/health/pregnancy/PR00122>

[56] *Risk Factors Present Before Pregnancy.* Merck Manual Home Edition. 1 February 2003. Accessed 19 May 2006 <http://www.merck.com/mmhe>

[57] Schuman, Andrew "A Concise History of Infant Formula (twists and turns included)" *Contemporary Pediatrics* 2003; 2:91

[58] Shuman, Tracy, "Depression and Pregnancy," *WebMD*, November 2005. Accessed 10 September 2006 <http://www.webmd.com/content/Article/51/40812.htm>

[59] "Tuskegee Syphilis Study" *Wikipedia* 3 May 2006. Accessed 18 May 2006 <http://en.wikipedia.org/wiki/tuskegee syphilis study>

[60] U.S. Consumer Products Safety Commission. Crib Safety Tips <www.cpsc.gov>

[61] US Department of Health and Human Services, Office on Women's Health, "An Easy Guide to Breastfeeding," May 2004

[62] Wesley, Joya, "Depression and African American Women," Black Women's Health. Accessed 10 September 2006. <www.blackwomenshealth.com>

[63] Westin, W.L. and Lane, Alfred T. *Color Textbook of Pediatric Dermatology*. Saint Louis: Mosby Year Book 1991

Index

A

Acrocyanosis, 134
Alcohol, 26, 61, 274
Anemia
    Diagnosis, 226
    Risk factors, 225
    Treatment, 226
Asthma, 33

B

Baby Necessities, 58
    Bassinette, 59, 103, 116, 242, 244
    Bath supplies, 61
    Changing pad, 59
    Changing table, 59
    Crib, 58
    Diapers and wipes, 63
    Infant basin, 60
    Infant carriers, 65
Baby powder, 61
Baby-proofing, 253
Bath supplies, 61
    Bath thermometer, 64
Bedding Supplies, 64
    Crib mattress, 65
Bed-sharing, 242, 243
Bilirubin, 99
Blood Sugar
    low, 97
Bottles
    Sterilization, 71
Bowel movements, 148
Bow-legs, 175
Breastfeeding Benefits
    Colostrum, 79
    Ovarian and Breast Cancer, 78
Breastfeeding Support
    African-American Breastfeeding Alliance, 70
    La Leche League, 70, 80, 262, 264

C

Car Safety, 55
    Harness system, 56
    LATCH, 55
    Locking clip, 55
Chest
    Accessory nipple, 198
    Breast buds, 198
Child care
    Certification, 252
    NAEYC, 252
Choking hazards, 66
Chronic Medical Conditions, 29
    Asthma, 29, 33
    Depression, 36, 122, 263, 274, 281, 282
    Diabetes, 29, 30, 274
    High Blood Pressure, 29, 31
    Lupus, 29, 33, 279
    Sarcoidosis, 29, 34, 35, 278
    Sickle Cell Anemia, 32, 220, 278
    Uterine Fibroids, 35
Circumsion, 231
Comforters, 64
Coming home
    First weeks
        Hair care, 119
        Skin care, 117
            Umbilical cord, 118

Sleeping, 114
Visitors, 111
Constipation, 202
Consumer Product Safety
  Commission, 52, 53,
  54, 262, 275
Co-sleeping, 242, 278
Cradle cap, 217
Crawling, 163
Crib Dangers
  Comforters, 64
  Stuffed toys, 64, 252,
    253
Crib safety
  Crib specifications, 54
Crying, 236, 237, 264
  Colic, 233
  Normal patterns, 237
  Reasons, 238

D

Depression, 36, 122, 263,
  274, 281, 282
Development
  2 months, 138
  4 months, 150
  6 months, 157
  9 months, 166
  One year, 172
Diabetes, 30, 274
  Gestational diabetes,
    29, 31
  Insulin, 30
  Type I, 30
  Type II, 30
Diarrhea, 201

E

Ears
  Ear infection, 185
  Ear pits and tags, 184
Eczema, 215
Exercise

Pregnancy and, 24
Extra digits
  Fingers, 207
  Toes, 207
Eyes
  Crossed-eyes, 180
  Eye color, 183
  Eye hemorrhages, 180
  Narrow tear duct, 181
  Pink-eye, 182
  Vision, 179

F

Feeding
  2 months, 145
  4 months, 153
  6 months, 158
  9 months, 167
  Breastfeeding, 79
    Contraindications,
      83
    Returning to work,
      82
  Formula Feeding, 83
    Preparation, 85
    Wet nurses, 83
  Low-iron formula, 203
  One year, 173
Feeding supplies, 70
  Bibs, 82
  Bottle warmers, 71
  Bottles, 71
  Breast pump, 70
  Commercial sterilizers,
    71
  Nipples, 71
Fetal Alcohol Syndrome,
  26
Fevers
  Height of, 255
  Newborn, 256
  Seizures, 258
  Treatment, 259

G

G6PD deficiency, 223
Growth charts, 131

H

Head, Eyes, Ear, Nose and throat
  Birth marks
    Eye, 183
  Caput and Cephalohematoma, 178
  Crossed-eyes, 180
  Ear infection, 185
  Ear pits and tags, 184
  Eye color, 183
  Eye hemorrhages, 180
  Narrow tear duct, 181
  Pink-eye, 182
  Positional molding, 179
Healthy Living, 22
Healthy People 2010, 14
Heart murmur, 219
Hernia
  Females, 235
  Males, 234
Hiccups, 134
Hospital stay
  Delivery room, 102
  First 24 hours, 105
  Going home, 109
    Car seat, 109
  Newborn hearing screen, 109
  Rooming-in, 107
  Second 24 hours, 107
  Vaccines, 105

I

Infant carriers, 65
Infant safety
  Walkers, 68

Infectious Diseases, 38, 40, 268, 269, 270
  Bacterial Vaginosis, 44
  Chickenpox, 49, 140, 173
  Gonorrhea and Chlamydia, 39
  Group B Streptococcus, 43, 44, 98
  Hepatitis B, 39, 105, 140, 152, 265, 269
  Herpes, 47
  HIV, 44, 45, 46, 83, 232, 272
  Listeriosis, 269
  Non-Routine Tests, 44
  Routine Tests, 48, 44
  Rubella, 43, 140, 173, 269
  Syphilis, 40, 41, 268, 281
  Trichomoniasis, 45

L

Laryngomalacia, 193
Lead
  History, 228
  Prevention, 230
Legs
  Positional molding, 206
Lungs
  Bronchiolitis, 194
    Albuterol, 196
Lupus, 33, 279

M

Medical Care
  Family Medicine, 76
  General Pediatrics, 76

Mouth
  Cysts, 188
  Teething, 188
  Thrush, 190
  Tooth Decay, 191

N

National Highway Transportation Safety Administration, 55, 262
Neck
  Torticollis, 193
Newborn period
  Delivery room
    Eye ointment, 104
    Vitamin K, 104
  Meconium, 107
  Newborn screen, 108
  Problems, 99
    Infection, 98
    Jaundice, 99
    Low blood sugar, 97
    Prematurity, 94
  Temperature control, 106
  Urine, 106
Nose
  Congestion, 187
  Milia, 187

P

Pets, 248
Postpartum check, 120
Postpartum depression, 122
Preparing for baby
  Car safety, 55
  Crib safety, 53, 281
  Hospital bag, 92
  Support system
    Mocha Moms, 87

R

Reflux, 204
  Silent, 205
Rickets, 272
  Vitamin D, 147

S

Safety
  Bathtub, 60
Sarcoidosis, 34, 35, 278
Separation anxiety, 169
Siblings, 245
Sickle Cell Anemia, 32, 220, 278
Skin
  Baby acne, 211
  Birth marks
    Café-au-lait, 212
    Mongolian spots, 213
  Diaper rashes
    Irritant, 213
    Yeast, 214
  Newborn rashes
    Congenital pustular melanosis, 210
  Skin color, 207
    Melanocytes, 208
  Sunblock, 209
Smoking, 24
Spoiling, 153
Stuffed toys, 64, 252, 253
Sudden infant death syndrome
  African-Americans, 241
  Back-to-Sleep, 241

T

Teething, 169
Toys, 66, 247
  Books, 69
Trimesters, 22

Types of delivery
   Assisted vaginal birth, 93
   Caesarean birth, 93

U

Umbilical cord, 135
Umbilical hernia, 200
Urinary tract infection, 233

V

Vaccines
   2 months, 139
   4 months, 152
   6 months, 163
   9 months, 167
   Concerns, 142
   Newborn, 134
   One year, 173
Vomiting, 199

W

Walking, 174
Well baby exam, 127
   2 months, 137
   6 months, 156
   4 months, 149
   9 months, 165
   One year, 171

www.ingramcontent.com/pod-product-compliance
Lightning Source LLC
Chambersburg PA
CBHW022053160426
43198CB00008B/215